Menstrual Problems for the MRCOG and Beyond

Second Edition

Published titles in the MRCOG and Beyond series

Antenatal Disorders for the MRCOG and Beyond
by Andrew Thomas and Ian Greer

Early Pregnancy Issues for the MRCOG and Beyond
by Geeta Kumar and Bidyut Kumar

Fetal Medicine for the MRCOG and Beyond, second edition
by Alan Cameron, Janet Breannand, Lena Crichton and Janice Gibson

Gynaecological and Obstetric Pathology for the MRCOG and Beyond, second edition
edited by Michael Wells, C Hilary Buckley and Harold Fox, with a chapter on cervical cytology by John Smith

Gynaecological Oncology for the MRCOG and Beyond, second edition
edited by Nigel Acheson and David Luesley

Haemorrhage and Thrombosis for the MRCOG and Beyond
edited by Anne Harper

Intrapartum Care for the MRCOG and Beyond, second edition
by Thomas F Baskett and Sabaratnam Arulkumaran, with a chapter on neonatal resuscitation by Gareth J Richards and a chapter on perinatal loss by Austin Ugwumadu and Melanie O'Byrne

Management of Infertility for the MRCOG and Beyond, second edition
edited by Siladitya Bhattacharya and Mark Hamilton

Medical Genetics for the MRCOG and Beyond
by Michael Connor

Menopause for the MRCOG and Beyond, second edition
by Margarat Rees

Neonatology for the MRCOG
by Peter Dear and Simon Newell

Paediatric and Adolescent Gynaecology for the MRCOG and Beyond, second edition
by Anne Garden, Mary Hernan and Joanne Topping

Psychological Disorders in Obstetrics and Gynaecology for the MRCOG and Beyond
by Khaled MK Ismail, Ilana Crome and PM Shaughn O'Brien

Reproductive Endocrinology for the MRCOG and Beyond, second edition
edited by Adam Balen

Urogynaecology for the MRCOG and Beyond, second edition
by Natalia Price and Simon Jackson

Menstrual Problems for the MRCOG and Beyond

Second Edition

Mary Ann Lumsden

and

Margaret Rees

CAMBRIDGE
UNIVERSITY PRESS

CAMBRIDGE
UNIVERSITY PRESS

University Printing House, Cambridge CB2 8BS, United Kingdom

Published in the United States of America by Cambridge University Press, New York

Cambridge University Press is part of the University of Cambridge.

It furthers the University's mission by disseminating knowledge in the pursuit of education, learning and research at the highest international levels of excellence.

www.cambridge.org
Information on this title: www.cambridge.org/9781107677388

First published 2014

Printed in Spain by Grafos SA Arte sobre papel

A catalogue record for this publication is available from the British Library

Library of Congress Cataloguing in Publication data
Lumsden, Mary Ann, author.
[Menstrual problems for the MRCOG]
Menstrual problems for the MRCOG and beyond / Mary Ann Lumsden, Margaret Rees. – Second edition.
p. ; cm. – (MRCOG and beyond series)
Includes bibliographical references and index.
ISBN 978-1-107-67738-8 (Paperback)
I. Rees, Margaret (Margaret C. P.), author II. Royal College of Obstetricians and Gynaecologists (Great Britain), issuing body. III. Title. IV. Series: MRCOG and beyond series.
[DNLM: 1. Menstruation Disturbances. WP 550]
RG163
618.1′72–dc23
2013047500

ISBN 978-1-107-67738-8 Paperback

Additional resources for this publication at www.cambridge.org/9781107677388

Contents

Abbreviations

ALA	aminolevulinic acid
AMH	anti-Müllerian hormone
ASRM	American Society for Reproductive Medicine
BEPS	benign edematous polysynovitis
BMI	body mass index
CBT	cognitive behavioural therapy
COC	combined oral contraceptive
COX	cyclooxygenase
CPP	chronic pelvic pain
D&C	dilatation and curretage
DUB	dysfunctional menstrual bleeding
ELA	endometrial laser ablation
ELITT™	endometrial laser intrauterine thermotherapy
FAI	free androgen index
FDA	US Food and Drug Administration
FSH	follicle-stimulating hormone
GnRH	gonadotrophin-releasing hormone
GP	general practitioner
HMB	heavy menstrual bleeding
HRT	hormone replacement therapy
ISPMD	International Society for Premenstrual Disorders
IUCD	intrauterine contraceptive device
IUS	intrauterine system
IVF	in vitro fertilization
LAVH	laparoscopic-assisted vaginal hysterectomy
LH	luteinizing hormone
LNG	levonorgestrel

LNG-IUS	levonorgestrel-releasing intrauterine system
LUNA	laparoscopic uterosacral nerve ablation
MEA®	microwave endometrial ablation
MRI	magnetic resonance imaging
NICE	National Institute for Health and Care Excellence
NSAID	nonsteroidal anti-inflammatory drug
PCOS	polycystic ovary syndrome
PID	pelvic inflammatory disease
PMDD	premenstrual dysphoric disorder
PMS	premenstrual syndrome
PMT	premenstrual tension
POF	premature ovarian failure
RBEA	rollerball endometrial ablation
SHBG	sex hormone-binding globulin
SSRI	selective serotonin reuptake inhibitor
STI	sexually transmitted infection
TCRE	transcervical resection of the endometrium
TENS	transcutaneous electrical nerve stimulation
UAE	uterine artery embolization

Preface

Menstrual problems are very common and thus it is essential that both trainees and consultants have a thorough knowledge of their investigation and treatment. Possession of the MRCOG is an essential component of specialist training within our specialty, both in the United Kingdom and in many countries overseas – the MRCOG has a high standing not only in the UK and the Commonwealth but increasingly within Europe. At the present time there are Fellows and Members of our College in over 80 countries throughout the world and the number of candidates taking the MRCOG examination continues to rise.

Preparing for the examination involves not only working in carefully monitored training posts but also a substantial amount of preparation related to research and clinical practice. In carrying out such studies candidates have traditionally used major standard works ranging from 'Jeffcoate's' and 'Donald' in days gone by to the present large, multi-author textbooks and the internet, the latter carrying information of variable quality.

Whilst the use of such sources is likely to continue as candidates quite rightly appreciate the comprehensive nature of them and the invaluable source references contained therein, in the 1990s, the Publications Committee of the Royal College of Obstetricians and Gynaecologists felt there was a need for a series of smaller, cheaper and more regularly updated texts on particular topics which need to be revised for the examination and would also be useful to those who have completed it. This book has now been thoroughly revised for the second time in order to maintain its relevance.

Patients with menstrual problems make up approximately one-third of the total number of women referred for outpatient gynaecological consultation. For that reason alone this is obviously a very important book – it is also important in that following decades of relative neglect basic scientists and clinical researchers are now taking a great deal of interest in the pathophysiology and possible new approaches to management for these common and distressing problems. This book has been written by one such team and will provide both an invaluable revision text and a most useful means of updating for practising clinicians.

Editors

Professor Mary Ann Lumsden MD, FRCOG,
Professor of Medical Education and Gynaecology,
University of Glasgow, and Honorary Consultant Gynaecologist,
Glasgow Royal Infirmary, Glasgow

Professor Margaret Rees MA, DPhil, FRCOG
Reader Emeritus in Reproductive Medicine, University of Oxford;
Visiting Professor, Faculty of Medicine, University of Glasgow; and
Adjunct Associate Professor, Robert Wood Johnson Medical School,
at Rutgers University New Brunswick, New Jersey

Contributors

Dr Jane Moore, MD, MRCOG
Honorary Consultant in Obstetrics and Gynaecology, Senior Fellow, Nuffield Department of Obstetrics and Gynaecology, University of Oxford

Dr Oliver Milling-Smith, MD, MRCOG
Consultant and Obstetrician and Gynaecologist,
Forth Valley NHS, Forth Valley Royal Hospital, Larbert, Scotland

Dr Stuart Jack MD, MSc, MRCOG
Consultant Obstetrician and Gynaecologist,
Aberdeen Royal Infirmary, Scotland

Dr Justin Clarke, MD, MRCOG
Consultant Obstetrician and Gynaecologist,
Birmingham Women's Hospital, Birmingham

1 Introduction

Menstrual problems are among the most common causes for GP and specialist referral, frequently accounting for one-third of gynaecological outpatient workload. The importance of menstrual disorder was acknowledged when the National Institute for Health and Care Excellence (NICE) commissioned a guideline on heavy menstrual bleeding (HMB), which was published in 2007.[1] Problems with menstruation are important since women today experience many more menstrual cycles during their reproductive life than they would have done 50 years ago. This is attributable to the fact that they have fewer pregnancies and also spend less time lactating. The average woman these days may expect 400 menstrual cycles in contrast to 40 in Victorian times.[2]

Women's lifestyles have also altered and it is not acceptable to suggest that menstrual problems are purely the woman's lot in life. Heavy periods can cause considerable inconvenience and are quite incompatible with the busy lifestyles of many women, who now expect swift and effective treatment for their problems.

It is of interest that the most common treatments vary from one country to another; in Sweden, for example, a woman's lifetime risk of having a hysterectomy performed is 12% whereas in parts of the USA it may be as high as 50%. Swedish women visit a gynaecologist with the expectation of receiving medical treatment; in many other parts of the western world they would expect a hysterectomy. This has considerable economic implications as well as suggesting that health education differs considerably around the world.

It is important that all gynaecologists have a basic understanding of menstrual reproductive physiology. This enables them to counsel women accurately and safely. Reassurance that there is no sinister pathology causing the problem is often all that is required, but such advice can only be given after appropriate investigation. Gynaecologists must also be in a position to offer up-to-date and appropriate treatment, which requires a thorough knowledge of the full range of options available. Some obtain information from guidelines either produced locally or nationally (for example, *Heavy Menstrual Bleeding* published by NICE).[1]

This book discusses the aetiology of menstrual problems, their presentation and investigation as well as medical and surgical management. Specific problems such as fibroid-associated bleeding, adolescent and perimenopausal bleeding and breakthrough bleeding are covered, as are other critically important problems such as premenstrual disorders, pelvic pain and dysmenorrhoea. The individual chapters have been produced by those with a particular interest in the area who are also practising clinicians and thus have first-hand experience.

Terminology

Research into menstrual disorders has been complicated by geographical variation in the definition of commonly used terms that mean one thing in the USA and another in the UK, the term menorrhagia being a good example. This means that 'heavy menstrual bleeding' should be used instead of 'menorrhagia' as it describes the symptom and everyone knows what is meant, making it easier to compare studies. This topic was the subject of a recent workshop and is discussed at greater length in Chapter 2.[3] The new terminology is becoming more accepted although inevitably it will take time.

Presentation

HEAVY MENSTRUAL BLEEDING (HMB)

The most common presenting menstrual problem is HMB. This complaint often follows a change in the woman's menstrual loss with an increase in flow which may have occurred relatively rapidly, or may have taken place over a number of years. It is difficult to assess the heaviness of flow clinically. It is well known that there is no correlation between the number of towels and tampons used and menstrual blood loss assessed objectively.[4] It may be more appropriate to ascertain the degree of incapacity experienced, in that some women are unable to leave the house for 1 or 2 days each month because of the heaviness of menstrual flow, whereas others are less inconvenienced.[5]

HMB is defined in the NICE Guideline as follows: **'Bleeding that interferes with a woman's physical, social, emotional and/or material quality of life.'**[1]

'Flooding' may lead to significant problems particularly if it is sudden and unexpected; thus, some women who actually have a blood loss within the normal range and are not compromised from a health point of view are seriously inconvenienced. Passage of clots causes concern for many women as this is perceived as abnormal. A pictorial assessment chart has been developed for the assessment of menstrual loss, although it has not achieved widespread acceptability.[6] However, it is very useful where objective evaluation is required.

MEASUREMENT OF MENSTRUAL BLOOD LOSS[8]

Investigations may be minimal in young women and hysterectomy must be virtually the only major operation carried out with no objective assessment of the problem. Blood loss can be measured easily but this is rarely done outside research projects, as collecting sanitary protection is not acceptable for many women. When blood loss is measured it yields fascinating information as it highlights those women whose problem is unlikely to have a physical basis, i.e. those complaining of HMB who have a menstrual blood loss of just a few millilitres. These women obviously have a problem but surgery may not be the most appropriate treatment for them. Measurement of haemoglobin is essential although menstrual problems can exist in the absence of anaemia. An assay of serum ferritin may be helpful.

A woman's approach to her periods will vary through her reproductive life. After childbearing is completed, the view of the menses will alter dramatically. 'Menstrual intolerance' is a phrase that has been coined to describe those who simply want an end to their periods. This may be said in a rather derogatory fashion, but for the reasons described in the first paragraph it is probably quite understandable.

INTERMENSTRUAL INTERVAL (CYCLE LENGTH)

Women perceive a decrease in inter-menstrual interval as abnormal, although this is not the case (Figure 1.1). The longest intermenstrual interval occurs at the menarche; regular periods then tend to be established until a woman reaches her 30s, when the intermenstrual interval is likely to shorten.[7] This is quite natural and the woman should be assured that there is nothing wrong with this (see Chapter 2 for a discussion of polymenorrhoea).

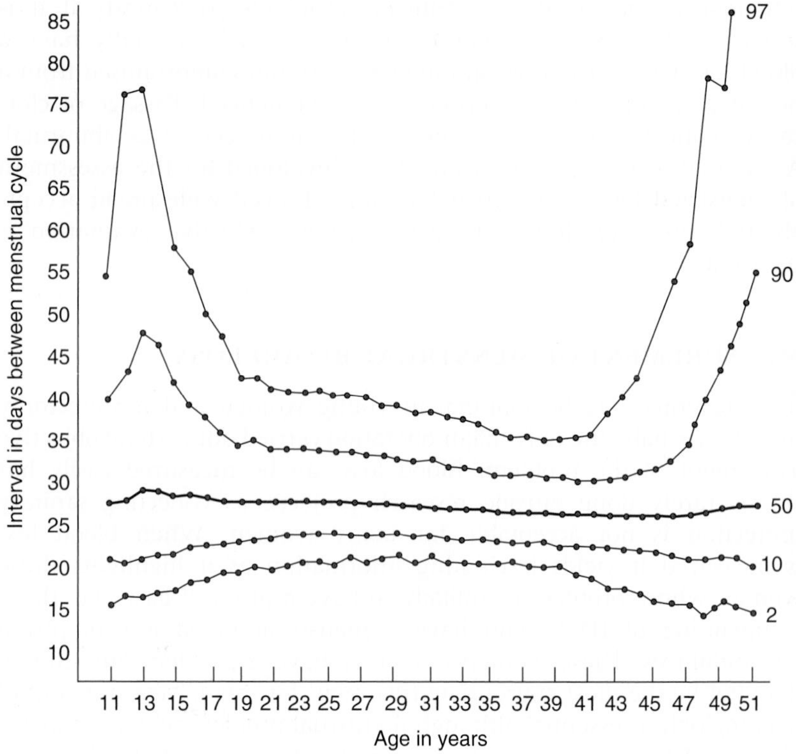

Figure 1.1 Menstrual cycles throughout the reproductive years; data from Treolar et al., 1967[7]

MENSTRUAL IRREGULARITY

Menstrual irregularity is a considerable nuisance for women because it leads to an unpredictable menstrual flow. It is most likely to occur at the extremes of reproductive life, the incidence of anovulation increasing as the menopause approaches. At the menopause unopposed estrogen production leads to persistent proliferative endometrium and occasionally hyperplastic change. This may be associated with extremely heavy bleeding at irregular intervals. Recently the menstrual cycle length has been used to predict the time and stage of the menopause.[9]

DYSMENORRHOEA

Dysmenorrhoea, or painful periods, may occur alone as the sole symptom in young, nulliparous women, or it may occur in conjunction with other menstrual problems, particularly in the older woman. Menstrual pain can be extremely debilitating, although overall the success rate for treatment is high. Division of dysmenorrhoea into primary and secondary is useful for the purposes of discussion although it can often be difficult to distinguish the two types on symptoms alone. Classical primary spasmodic dysmenorrhoea occurs at the onset of the menses and gets better after 1 or 2 days, whereas secondary dysmenorrhoea tends to start prior to the menses and worsens as it proceeds. However, there is considerable overlap between these two groups.

Any menstrual problem may be associated with premenstrual syndrome, although this is not discussed at length in this book. Premenstrual syndrome can often be successfully treated by therapies inducing anovulation. Many symptoms can be clustered premenstrually, including irritability, loss of concentration and emotional liability, as well as premenstrual headache, migraine and even epileptic fits. The treatment for these problems is particularly problematical, with no one specific treatment being successful.

ABNORMAL MENSTRUATION

The defects considered here are HMB and other menstrual abnormalities not particularly associated with infertility as the principal complaint, although endometriosis, fibroids and polycystic ovarian syndrome may be exceptions.

References

1. National Institute for Health and Clinical Excellence. *Heavy Menstrual Bleeding*. NICE clinical guideline 44. London: NICE; 2007.
2. Rees MCP, Turnbull AC. Menstrual disorders – an overview. *Baillieres Clin Obstet Gynaecol* 1989;3:217–26.
3. Fraser IS, Critchley HO, Broder M, Munro MG. The FIGO recommendations on terminologies and definitions for normal and abnormal uterine bleeding. *Semin Reprod Med* 2011;29:383–90.
4. Chimbira TH, Anderson AB, Turnbull AC. Relation between measured menstrual blood loss and patient's subjective assessment of loss, duration of bleeding, number of sanitary towels used, uterine weight and endometrial surface area. *Br J Obstet Gynaecol* 1980;87:603–9.
5. Warner PE, Critchley HO, Lumsden MA, Campbell-Brown M, Douglas A, Murray GD. Menorrhagia I: measured blood loss, clinical features, and outcomes in women with heavy periods: a survey with follow-up data. *Am J Obstet Gynecol* 2004;190:1216–23.
6. Higham JM, O'Brien PM, Shaw RW. Assessment of menstrual blood loss using a pictorial chart. *Br J Obstet Gynaecol* 1990;97:734–9.

7. Treolar AE, Boynton RE, Behn BG, Brown DW. Variation of the human menstrual cycle through reproductive life. *Int J Fertil* 1967;12:77–126.
8. Fraser IS, McGarron G, Markham R, Resta T, Watts A. Measured menstrual blood loss in women with pelvic disease or coagulation disorder. *Obstet Gynecol* 1986;68:630–3.
9. Harlow SD, Gass M, Hall JE, Lobo R, Maki P, Rebar RW, et al.; STRAW + 10 Collaborative Group. Executive summary of the Stages of Reproductive Aging Workshop + 10: addressing the unfinished agenda of staging reproductive aging. *Menopause* 2012;19:387–95.

2 Excessive menstrual bleeding

Excessive menstrual bleeding describes the clinical problems of heavy menstrual blood loss together with frequent or irregular menstruation. It is important that all gynaecologists have a basic understanding of menstrual reproductive physiology. This enables them to counsel patients accurately and safely. Reassurance that there is no sinister pathology causing the problem is often all that is required, but such advice can only be given after appropriate investigation. Gynaecologists must also be in a position to offer up-to-date and appropriate treatment, requiring a thorough knowledge of the full range of options available. This chapter addresses endometrial morphology, the mechanism of menstruation and the aetiology and management of menstrual problems.

Endometrial morphology

The human endometrium is a dynamic tissue that, in response to the prevailing steroid environment of sequential ovarian estrogen and progesterone exposure, undergoes well-characterized cycles of proliferation, differentiation and tissue breakdown on a monthly basis. If pregnancy fails to be established then the upper two-thirds of the endometrium (functional layer) is shed via menstruation. Endometrial regeneration then occurs from the basal layer.

There are three well-characterized phases of endometrial development: a preovulatory **proliferative** phase; a postovulatory **secretory** phase; and a **menstrual** phase involving tissue breakdown.

Endometrial dating has historically been related to the timing of ovulation. The series of classical morphological changes that occur in response to cyclical ovarian activity have been well detailed.[1] However, much controversy surrounds endometrial dating and some arguments suggest that histological dating, according to traditional histological methods, lacks both the accuracy and precision to provide a guide for clinical management. More robust methods for endometrial dating are likely to involve combining histological dating with reporting of last menstrual period and quantification of circulating estrogen and progesterone levels. Detailed gene microarray studies support this method for characterizing endometrial samples with consistency across these three parameters.[2]

It is also notable that exogenous administration of steroids produces a deviation from the classical histological features of glandular structure, mitotic status of glandular cells and secretions in the lumen of the glands[3] when compared with accurately dated endometrium collected during a physiological cycle.

Mechanism of menstruation

The menstrual cycle is clinically described according to its regularity and duration of bleeding. The average length between menses is between 21 and 35 days with the duration of bleeding lasting 4–5 days.

During the luteal (secretory) stage of the menstrual cycle, in the absence of fertilization, there is regression of the corpus luteum, leading to a decline of the steroid hormone, progesterone. During the secretory phase, prior to this decline in circulating hormone levels, there is already a decline of endometrial sex steroid receptor expression in the superficial layer of the endometrium. The epithelial glands within the superficial layer of the endometrium are negative in their immunostaining for progesterone and estrogen receptors. It is therefore hypothesized that the declining levels of steroids can only be directly detected in the stromal cells of the superficial layer, which persistently stain for progesterone receptors.[4] Additional evidence has demonstrated that menstruation can be blocked by progesterone add-back up to 36 hours after steroid decline.[5] It would therefore appear that menstruation specifically occurs in response to the decline of progesterone levels.

In 1940, Markee[6] was able to perform classical studies into the mechanism of menstruation. By transplanting explants of human endometrial tissue into the anterior chamber of a Rhesus monkey's eye, they were able to visualize direct events that occurred in response to progesterone withdrawal. In response to steroid decline, they observed stromal shrinkage, increased coiling of spiral arterioles and vascular stasis. These changes were followed by a period of vasodilation and perivascular bleeding and 24 hours later, a subsequent intense vasoconstriction and tissue necrosis prior to menstruation itself.

The molecular mechanism of menstruation in response to progesterone withdrawal is a complex cascade of events that have yet to be fully elucidated. It in part involves the production of prostaglandins that are able to induce vasoconstriction leading to a reduced blood flow to the endometrium. Subsequently there is increased expression of a range of locally acting mediators including cytokines, angiogenic

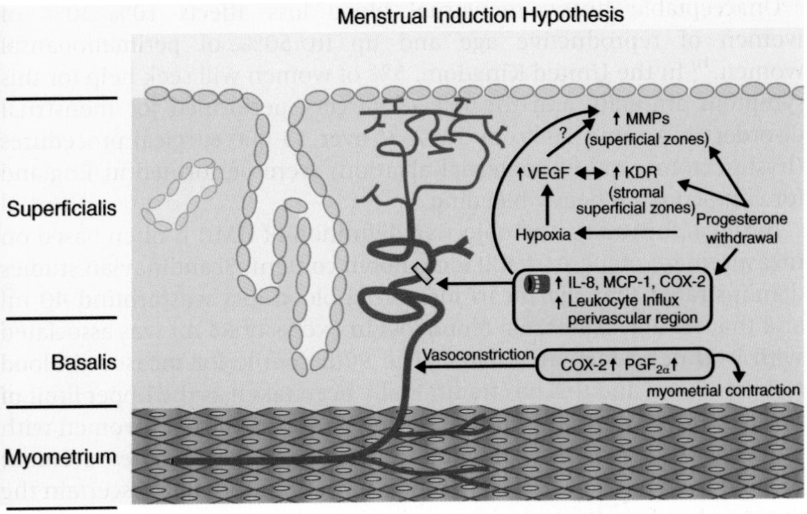

Figure 2.1 Hypothetical mechanism of menstruation. Adapted from Critchley, Kelly, Brenner, Baird. 2001 *Clin. Endocrinol.* 55: 701 –10[7]

factors, protease enzymes and further prostaglandins. The cumulative endpoint of these changes in local mediators, together with an influx of migratory leukocytes is the process of menstruation. Figure 2.1 illustrates the hypothetical mechanism of menstruation.[7]

Coincident events of progesterone withdrawal and hypoxia Progesterone withdrawal results in an up-regulation of inflammatory mediators, production of matrix metalloproteinases and a leukocyte influx in the upper endometrial zones. There is coincident hypoxia and an up-regulation of matrix metalloproteinase production in the same endometrial upper zone stromal cells. Menstrual sloughing takes place from the superficial regions of the endometrium.

Aetiology of excessive menstrual bleeding

HEAVY MENSTRUAL BLEEDING

Menorrhagia is a clinical definition describing heavy menstrual blood loss. Heavy menstrual bleeding (HMB) has been accepted internationally as a more accurate terminology for this condition.[8] This term shall be used in preference to menorrhagia during the rest of this section. HMB is defined as excessive menstrual blood loss, which can interfere with a woman's physical, social, emotional and/or material quality of life.[9]

Unacceptable heavy menstrual blood loss affects 10%–30% of women of reproductive age and up to 50% of perimenopausal women.[10] In the United Kingdom, 5% of women will seek help for this symptom annually and the risk of surgery performed for menstrual disorders is around 20%. In 2002–3, over 13 000 surgical procedures (hysterectomy and endometrial ablation) were performed in England for complaints of heavy bleeding.[11]

In research studies, the objective definition of HMB is often based on measurement of menstrual haemoglobin content. Scandinavian studies demonstrated that the mean menstrual blood loss was around 40 ml and that regular menstrual blood loss in excess of 63 ml was associated with iron deficiency anaemia.[12] The 90th centile for measured blood loss was 80 ml and this has traditionally been taken as the upper limit of normal. However, in the clinical setting only 40%–60% of women with perceived heavy menstrual blood loss have an objective measurement of greater than 80 ml.[13] It is therefore more appropriate to ascertain the degree of incapacity experienced, in that some women are unable to leave the house for 1 or 2 days each month because of the heaviness of menstrual flow, whereas others are less inconvenienced. 'Flooding' may lead to significant problems, particularly if it is sudden and unexpected; thus some women who actually have a blood loss within the normal range and are not compromised from a health point of view are seriously inconvenienced. Passage of clots cause concern to many women, as this is perceived as abnormal. A pictorial chart has been developed for the assessment of menstrual loss, although it has not achieved widespread acceptability.[14] It is, however, used in many clinical trials either in its original or modified form.

The classification of abnormal uterine bleeding

A new classification system for causes of abnormal uterine bleeding (AUB) in the reproductive years was developed by the International Federation of Gynaecology and Obstetrics in November 2010. The system is based on the acronym PALM-COEIN[15] that covers the causes of abnormal menstrual bleeding polyps, adenomyosis, leiomyoma, malignancy and hyperplasia, coagulopathy, ovulatory disorders, endometrial causes, iatrogenic. This novel classification was developed in response to concerns about the design and interpretation of basic science and clinical investigation that relates to the problem of abnormal uterine bleeding. This has led to much confusion when considering the results of clinical trials and also, methods of treating a particular problem, e.g. 'menorrhagia' meant different things on the two sides of the Atlantic and has now been replaced with Heavy Menstrual Bleeding.

A system of nomenclature for the description of normal uterine bleeding and the various symptoms that comprise abnormal bleeding has also been included. The new nomenclature also enhances education and communication between clinicians and scientists, which should improve our understanding and management of this often perplexing clinical condition.

A very common cause relates to ovulatory dysfunction, which typically leads to a combination of irregular bleeding and a variable volume of menstrual flow, which can lead to HMB. In the past this was thought to be the principle reason for ovulatory dysfunction but with improved scanning, more pathologies, e.g. fibroids, adenomyosis or polyps are being identified, which can be sub-classified further according to their position in the uterus. Most often, the woman is either not ovulating, has infrequent ovulation or, especially in the late reproductive years, has deficiency of luteal function. To be classified as having an ovulatory disorder, the individual should have a cycle length in the previous 6 months that varies by at least 21 days, although this may be subject to change with time.

HMB does occur in the presence of ovulation and apparent absence of organic pathology. There are no differences in histology, steroid hormone concentrations or steroid receptor concentrations. However, substantial evidence does exist implicating local mediators, in particular disturbances of arachidonic acid metabolism, disturbances of angiogenic processes or alterations in factors such as matrix metalloproteinases.[16] It appears that there may be a shift in endometrial prostaglandin signalling from the vasoconstrictor prostaglandins ($PGF_2\alpha$) to the vasodilator prostaglandins (PGE_2 or prostacyclin).

CLOTTING DISORDERS

Clotting disorders such as von Willebrand's disease are another cause of HMB.[17] Bleeding disorders are often thought to represent a small proportion of women presenting with heavy menstrual loss. However, studies have shown that 13% of women with HMB have a previously undiagnosed bleeding disorder of von Willebrand's disease.[18] Patients with platelet and coagulation disorders frequently suffer from heavy menstrual blood loss, necessitating hormonal or surgical therapy and sometimes blood transfusions. In women with thrombocytopenia, menstrual blood loss correlates broadly with platelet count at the time of the menses. Splenectomy has been known to reduce the menstrual blood loss in these patients dramatically.

Reduced clotting is a known feature at the time of menstruation.[19] However, there is no impairment of blood coagulation in those with heavy menstrual loss, nor are fibrin degradation products elevated in the menstrual fluid of those with heavy menstrual loss.

PELVIC PATHOLOGIES

HMB is thought to be associated with uterine fibroids, adenomyosis, pelvic infection, endometrial polyps and the presence of a foreign body such as an inert or copper-containing intrauterine contraceptive device (IUCD). However, objective evidence of HMB in most of these situations is remarkably limited. Pelvic pathologies such as fibroids are common, affecting between 20 and 25% of women. It is reported that around a third of women with fibroids complain of heavy menstrual blood loss. In women with menstrual blood loss greater than 200 ml per month, over half will have fibroids. Around 40% of those with adenomyosis have menstrual blood loss in excess of 80 ml per menses. Whether chronic pelvic inflammatory disease (PID) or endometrial polyps are associated with above-average loss is unclear. There is evidence for a role for prostaglandins in HMB associated with adenomyosis, uterine leiomyomata and the presence of an IUCD.[20] Endometrial production of vasodilator prostaglandins is raised in the presence of adenomyosis, and prostaglandin production is also increased in the presence of an IUCD. However, the non-steroidal anti-inflammatory drugs (NSAIDs) are less effective in HMB associated with IUCD presence than in DUB, making it likely that other factors are also important.

MEDICAL DISORDERS

HMB is associated with various endocrine disorders such as thyroid dysfunction and Cushing's disease, although the mechanisms are unknown.

Polymenorrhoea

Women perceive a decrease in intermenstrual interval as abnormal although this is not the case. The longest intermenstrual interval occurs at the menarche, regular periods then tend to be established until a woman reaches her 30s when the intermenstrual interval is likely to shorten. This is quite natural and the patient should be assured that there is nothing wrong with this. Polymenorrhoea is the term given to women who bleed too often either because of prolonged bleeding or because of a shortened intermenstrual interval. It is a term of limited application, an accurate description of the menstrual cycle is much more useful in the assessment of a woman's menstrual disturbance.

Management of menstrual complaints

There are a number of terminologies to describe menstrual complaints such as menorrhagia, polymenorrhoea, oligomenorrhoea, polymenorrhagia and metrorrhagia. Often these terms are not of value and may lead to clinical distraction from the patient's complaint. An accurate account of the menstrual cycle is preferable to avoid confusion. It is also important to listen to the patient, since many women are referred with 'heavy periods' when this is not their principal complaint. This means that the referral letters may be misleading, reinforcing the need to take an accurate history of the woman's menstrual complaint.

CLINICAL HISTORY

A careful history is mandatory, and should include details of: the length of bleeding; the length of the cycle (often best elicited by asking the interval between the first day of one period and the first day of the next); the number of heavy days of menstrual bleeding; the presence and number of days of any pain; and the incapacity caused by the period. If present, the duration of the pain should also be ascertained. Details of any irregular bleeding should be elicited, particularly inter-menstrual or postcoital bleeding, as well as pain occurring either during the menstrual bleed or with intercourse. These symptoms suggest other possible pathologies such as cervical pathology or endometriosis, taking the clinician down a different clinical pathway to HMB alone.

The patient may also complain of symptoms that are exacerbated by the menstrual period. Feeling tired is a common complaint that is not necessarily related to the presence of anaemia. Details of any previous treatments are important, together with their effectiveness and side effects. A majority of women will have had some form of medical treatment (whether appropriate or not) before coming to the gynaecological outpatients' clinic. It is also quite useful to establish at this stage the expectation of the patient as to what she is hoping the gynaecologist will be able to achieve. Some women simply require reassurance that they don't have malignant disease or that they are not going through the menopause at an inappropriate time. Others are very keen to have an end to their periods all together – this group is likely to opt for hysterectomy sooner or later. Many patients do not know that there are alternative options to hysterectomy. Although a large proportion of uteri removed at hysterectomy are normal in structure, it is important to remember that biochemical problems may be present within the uterus. These cannot be visualised by a pathologist or with the naked eye.

CLINICAL EXAMINATION AND INVESTIGATIONS

The NICE guideline on HMB gives clear guidance on examination and investigation, as outlined in the following paragraphs. In primary care management of HMB, if the history is not suggestive of a structural or histological abnormality, it is acceptable to omit a pelvic examination and start empirical medical treatment. However, symptoms such as inter-menstrual bleeding, postcoital bleeding, pelvic pain and/or pressure symptoms may suggest structural or histological pathologies associated with the patient's menstrual complaint. Treatment failures should also raise concerns about additional pathologies. These clinical situations warrant a physical examination, and recommendations suggest a physical examination is required in the following situations:[9]

- before all levonorgestrel-releasing intrauterine system (LNG-IUS) fittings
- before investigations for histological abnormalities
- before requesting a pelvic ultrasound scan.

Ultrasound is the first-line diagnostic tool for detecting structural abnormalities. It should be noted that an ultrasound examination should only be organized in the following situations:[9]

- the uterus is palpable abdominally
- the patient's build precludes an accurate examination
- a pelvic mass is suspected
- there has been a failure of medical treatment.

When there is a concern about possible histological abnormalities or in a woman over the age of 45, a biopsy should be taken to exclude endometrial carcinoma or atypical hyperplasia.

A full blood count should be carried out on all women with HMB. However, a serum ferritin test should not routinely be requested.

Testing for coagulation disorders such as von Willebrand's disease should be considered in younger women with HMB. Hormone profile tests are of no value and thyroid function tests should only be requested when other signs or symptoms of thyroid disease are present.

Treatment

Specific diseases may require particular measures depending on their nature. However, many cases of HMB are not associated with a particular disorder and can be treated medically or surgically, as described in Chapters 3 and 4.

References

1. Noyes RW, Hertig AT, Rock J. Dating the endometrial biopsy. *Fertil Steril* 1950;1:3–25.
2. Talbi S, Hamilton AE, Vo KC, et al. Molecular phenotyping of human endometrium distinguishes menstrual cycle phases and underlying biological processes in normo-ovulatory women. *Endocrinology* 2006;147:1097–121.
3. Habiba MA, Bell SC, Al-Azzawi F. Endometrial responses to hormone replacement therapy: histological features compared with those of late luteal phase endometrium. *Hum Reprod* 1998;13:1674–82.
4. Critchley HO, Brenner RM, Henderson TA, et al. Estrogen receptor beta, but not estrogen receptor alpha, is present in the vascular endothelium of the human and nonhuman primate endometrium. *J Clin Endocrinol Metab* 2001;86:1370–8.
5. Brenner RM, Nayak NR, Slayden OD, Critchley HO, Kelly RW. Premenstrual and menstrual changes in the macaque and human endometrium: relevance to endometriosis. *Ann N Y Acad Sci* 2002;955: 60–74; discussion 86, 396–406.
6. Markee JE. Menstruation in intraocular endometrial transplants in the rhesus monkey. *Contributions to Embryology* 1940;28:219–308.
7. Critchley HO, Kelly RW, Brenner RM, Baird DT. The endocrinology of menstruation – a role for the immune system. *Clin Endocrinol (Oxf)* 2001;55:701–10.
8. Fraser IS, Critchley HO, Munro MG, Broder M. Can we achieve international agreement on terminologies and definitions used to describe abnormalities of menstrual bleeding? *Hum Reprod* 2007;22:635–43.
9. National Institute for Health and Clinical Excellence. *Heavy Menstrual Bleeding: Investigation and Treatment*. Clinical guideline 44. London: NICE: 2007 [http://www.nice.org.uk/guidance/CG44].
10. Prentice A. Health burden of menstrual disorders. In: O'Brien S, Cameron I, MacLean A (editors). *Disorders of the Menstrual Cycle*. London: RCOG Press; 2000. pp. 171–86.
11. Reid PC, Virtanen-Kari S. Randomised comparative trial of the levonorgestrel intrauterine system and mefenamic acid for the treatment of idiopathic menorrhagia: a multiple analysis using total menstrual fluid loss, menstrual blood loss and pictorial blood loss assessment charts. *BJOG* 2005;112:1121–5.

12. Hallberg L, Hogdahl AM, Nilsson L, Rybo G. Menstrual blood loss – a population study. Variation at different ages and attempts to define normality. *Acta Obstet Gynecol Scand* 1966;45:320–51.
13. Fraser IS, Pearse C, Shearman RP, Elliott PM, McIlveen J, Markham R. Efficacy of mefenamic acid in patients with a complaint of menorrhagia. *Obstet Gynecol* 1981;58:543–51.
14. Higham JM, O'Brien PMS, Shaw RM. Assessment of menstrual blood loss using a pictorial chart. *Br J Obstet Gynaecol* 1990;97:734.
15. Munro MG, Critchley HO, Fraser IS. The FIGO systems for nomenclature and classification of causes of abnormal uterine bleeding in the reproductive years: who needs them? *Am J Obstet Gynecol* 2012;207:259–65.
16. Jabbour HN, Sales KJ, Smith OP, Battersby S, Boddy SC. Prostaglandin receptors are mediators of vascular function in endometrial pathologies. *Mol Cell Endocrinol* 2006;252:191–200.
17. Kouides PA. Obstetric and gynaecological aspects of von Willebrand disease. *Best Pract Res Clin Haematol* 2001;14:381–99.
18. Lukes AS, Kadir RA, Peyvandi F, Kouides PA. Disorders of hemostasis and excessive menstrual bleeding: prevalence and clinical impact. *Fertil Steril* 2005;84:1338–44.
19. Livingstone M, Fraser IS. Mechanisms of abnormal uterine bleeding. *Hum Reprod Update* 2002;8:60–7.
20. Fraser IS, McCarron G, Markham R, Resta T, Watts A. Measured menstrual blood loss in women with menorrhagia associated with pelvic disease or coagulation disorder. *Obstet Gynecol* 1986;68:630–3.

3 Investigation

The purpose of uterine cavity evaluation is to make an accurate diagnosis of the cause of abnormal uterine bleeding, in order that therapy can be appropriately tailored to the woman. The traditional approach to investigating menstrual problems was dilatation and curettage (D&C). However, since the mid-1980s, less invasive techniques have been developed to allow evaluation of the uterus and endometrium without the need for hospital admission or general anaesthesia. These diagnostic technologies include pelvic ultrasound, hysteroscopy and endometrial biopsy and have largely replaced the necessity for D&C. This chapter reviews the accuracy and efficacy of currently available tests used to evaluate the uterine cavity.

History and examination

All women presenting with menstrual problems should be evaluated initially with a full history and clinical examination. Since systemic disease, such as weight loss or hypo- or hyperthyroidism, may affect the menstrual pattern, it is important to consider the whole person and not just the reproductive tract. Menstrual problems can have a substantial adverse impact on health-related quality of life, so it is important to ascertain the degree to which menstrual symptoms are restricting a woman's activities of daily living and affecting her well-being.

A careful speculum and bimanual examination should be performed. This allows the lower genital tract and cervix to be inspected for abnormal areas and swabs to be taken for culture, where appropriate. Uterine size can be assessed on bimanual examination; if the uterus is greater in size than 12 weeks of gestation, it may be palpable abdominally. Do not forget that ovarian lesions can affect the menstrual pattern, although this is unusual. If an ovarian abnormality is suspected, ultrasound may be useful for further assessment. Blood loss is notoriously difficult to quantify from history alone. Menstrual blood loss can be quantified objectively by using the alkaline haematin method and involves the patient collecting menstrual pads. Semi-objective methods have been developed using various pictorial aids and are less burdensome. However, accurate measurement of menstrual loss is in general only necessary within a research context.

Amenorrhoea

Women with amenorrhoea (no menstrual bleeding for 6 months) should have a full history and examination as described above. If amenorrhoea is thought to be attributable to an abnormality of the uterine cavity, such as Asherman's syndrome, hysteroscopy may help in diagnosis.

Postmenopausal bleeding

Postmenopausal bleeding can be defined as vaginal bleeding after an absence of 12 months in women in whom the stock of ovarian follicles is exhausted. Women presenting with this complaint should have a full history and vaginal examination followed by formal investigation of the uterine cavity without delay.

Dilatation and curettage (D&C)

D&C used to be the method of choice for assessing the uterine cavity but, with the advent of uterine imaging and less invasive methods of obtaining endometrial tissue and samples, has now become a second-line test. Between 2000 and 2010, the annual number of D&C procedures declined from 30 000 to 8000.[1] The procedure involves dilatation of the cervical canal (usually under general anaesthesia) and curettage of the endometrial cavity. The endometrial curettings obtained are examined histologically.

D&C is still a common gynaecological procedure and is undoubtedly familiar to the reader. Details of the procedure can be found in *Rob & Smith's Operative Surgery: Gynaecology and Obstetrics*.[2]

EFFICACY

It was often assumed that careful D&C followed by histological examination of curettings will correctly identify all women with endometrial pathology. However, this is almost certainly not true, as demonstrated in studies comparing pathology of endometrium obtained at curettage with pathology of the uterus obtained at hysterectomy. In a study of 407 women, 33 of whom had adenocarcinoma, the diagnosis was missed in five (15%) women using D&C.[3] Other studies confirm these data, with reports of at least 5% of cases of endometrial carcinoma missed by D&C. These results are not surprising given that, when curettage is undertaken before hysterectomy, examination of the hysterectomy specimen indicates that less than 75% of the uterine cavity is curetted in the majority of women.

D&C also appears to be less sensitive than hysteroscopy for evaluation of the uterine cavity, particularly in the diagnosis of uterine fibroids and endometrial polyps.[4,5] This is discussed further in the section on hysteroscopy below.

SAFETY

The mortality rate associated with D&C is extremely low. However, the incidence of complications such as haemorrhage, perforation and infection ranges from 3/1000 to 13/1000. Up to 5/1000 women proceed unexpectedly to a major operation as a result of complications arising from D&C.[6]

BOX 3.1 KEY POINTS: D&C

D&C is:

- an established technique to obtain endometrial tissue for histological analysis
- indicated where outpatient tests to evaluate the uterus are inappropriate or have failed to make a diagnosis
- less effective than hysteroscopy and directed biopsy in the diagnosis of endometrial carcinoma
- associated with complications leading to further surgical intervention in up to 5/1000 procedures.

Hysteroscopy

Hysteroscopy is the visualization of the uterine cavity using a narrow, flexible or rigid telescope inserted through the cervix. Abnormal endometrium is visualized and confirmed by directed biopsy (Figure 3.1).

Hysteroscopy was first described by Pantaleoni in 1896. With improvements in fibre optics and televisual engineering, by the 1970s diagnostic hysteroscopy had become an accepted technique. However, hysteroscopy became widespread in UK gynaecological practice only after the realization that hysteroscopy facilitated intrauterine surgical procedures such as endometrial ablation.

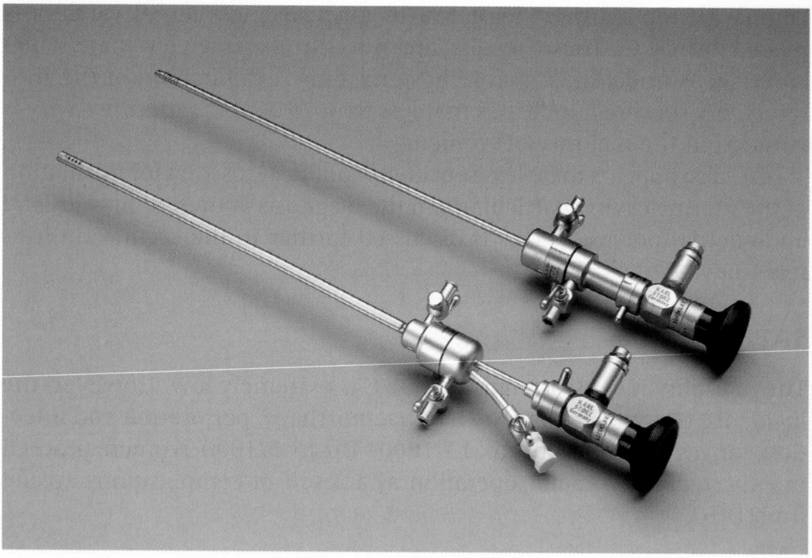

Figure 3.1 Hysteroscopes

EQUIPMENT

In the UK, hysteroscopy is usually carried out using a rigid hysteroscope consisting of a telescope within an outer sheath. This instrument gives a clear image and is relatively easy to use. The image can be viewed directly through the eyepiece, but the eyepiece should be coupled to a digital camera to enable display on a video screen. A video system has many advantages:

- other theatre staff, students and assistants can watch the procedure
- a permanent record of the operative findings can be made
- there are significant advantages in terms of comfort for the operator
- further magnification is achieved.

The terminal objective lens is set at either 0° or 30° to the area to be visualised. The 0° straightforward telescope provides vision from the normal perspective, thereby facilitating orientation and is therefore easiest to use. The advantage of a 30° terminal lens relates to increased field of view compared with a 0° lens, with rotation around the axis allowing panoramic viewing of all aspects of the uterus including more inaccessible areas such as tubal ostia. Light is conducted to the end of the hysteroscope by means of fibre optic light bundles.

Conventional hysteroscopes have a ×8 magnification system, although more detailed visualisation of the glandular structure of the endometrium is possible using more specialized hysteroscopes with higher magnification. However, these contact hysteroscopes are rarely used. An outer sheath, tightly coupled to the hysteroscope itself to prevent leakage, is required around the hysteroscope as a conduit for the passage of media to distend the uterus. The standard diagnostic hysteroscope used to be 4 mm in diameter enclosed in a 5 mm single flow outer sheath, thus allowing the procedure to be performed without recourse to cervical dilatation in the majority of women. However, advances in engineering and fibre optic technology have led to miniaturization of telescopes (1.0–2.9 mm) and, although the images are smaller and less bright, there is no significant compromise in image quality. Total working diameters of modern diagnostic systems are well under 5 mm (typically 2.5–4 mm). This has facilitated the use of no-touch vaginoscopy, where the entire procedure is performed without the use of a vaginal speculum or cervical instrumentation.[7] Operative hysteroscopy requires an integrated or additional sheath for outflow to provide continuous flow and irrigation of the uterine cavity. A working channel within the inflow sheath allows for passage of miniature ancillary mechanical and electrosurgical instruments, which are used to take directed biopsies and remove focal pathologies such as polyps.

A light source and cable and a source of distension medium complete the equipment. A xenon generator gives the best light with minimal heat generation, which is particularly important during operative hysteroscopy. The medium for distension of the uterus can be either gaseous, using carbon dioxide, or fluid. However, fluid is used predominantly because it facilitates operative interventions by continuously irrigating the cavity and does not require use of specialized pumps. A fluid-based medium, using physiological normal saline or glycine, is preferred for operative hysteroscopy. Where larger-diameter (8–10 mm) hysteroscopy systems such as resectoscopes are employed, the infusion of fluid distention medium should be controlled carefully because of the risk of fluid overload or gas embolus. A pump may aid continuous flow.

TECHNIQUE

Ideally, hysteroscopy should be performed in the proliferative phase (days 6–14) of the menstrual cycle because the endometrium is thinner and more regular, facilitating accurate diagnosis. The choice of anaesthesia depends on the procedure to be performed and the equipment available. For the majority of women, diagnostic hysteroscopy can be performed in an outpatient setting without anaesthesia. Minor operative procedures can also be performed in the same setting with recourse to local paracervical or direct cervical anaesthesia when cervical dilatation is required. General anaesthesia is indicated for operative interventions with larger-diameter hysteroscopes (over 6 mm), where outpatient procedures are not appropriate or have failed because of patient factors.

The standard approach to hysteroscopy was developed for the anaesthetized woman. The woman is placed in the lithotomy position and the perineum and vagina are cleansed. The operative area is then draped, the cervix grasped with a volsellum, the cervical canal dilated and the hysteroscope inserted into the uterus as far as the fundus, under direct vision. The widespread adoption of the outpatient setting has placed more emphasis on patient comfort. Miniature hysteroscopes are used and unnecessary manipulation or instrumentation of the lower genital tract is avoided. The RCOG Green-top Guideline *Best Practice in Outpatient Hysteroscopy* summarizes the evidence and delineates current best practice for outpatient hysteroscopy.[8] The uterine cavity is examined systematically by manipulation of the hysteroscope to provide panoramic and closer, magnified views. Maintenance of orientation is important, especially for operative interventions; this can be achieved by paying careful attention to the alignment of the camera and hysteroscope.

As the surgeon becomes familiar with the hysteroscopic appearance of the endometrium according to menopausal status and phase of the menstrual cycle, deviations from normal will become apparent (Figures 3.2 and 3.3). An abnormal endometrial appearance, suggestive of potentially premalignant hyperplastic or malignant disease, requires a representative confirmatory biopsy to be taken. This can be achieved by taking a hysteroscopically directed biopsy (which gives a very small sample for histology), outpatient global biopsy devices (such as the Pipelle-type biopsy) or formal D&C. Hysteroscopy is the gold standard test for diagnosing focal pathologies such as polyps, submucous fibroids, intrauterine adhesions and septa, and for the visualization and retrieval of lost intrauterine contraceptive devices.[8,9]

EFFICACY

Hysteroscopy combined with directed or global biopsy is normally performed to exclude serious endometrial pathology, mainly endometrial carcinoma, and also to diagnose and treat local minor pathology such as endometrial polyps.

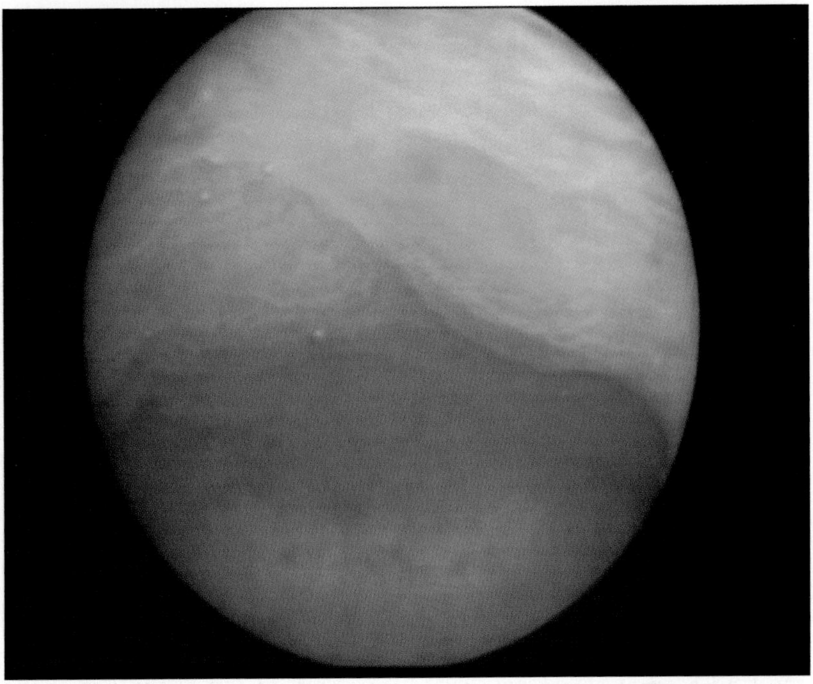

Figure 3.2 Secretory-phase endometrium at hysteroscopy

SAFETY

Complications of hysteroscopy include uterine perforation, cervical laceration and reaction to distension media. However, these complications are rare during diagnostic hysteroscopy using no or local anaesthesia and the procedure is probably safer than conventional curettage under general anaesthetic.[10]

HYSTEROSCOPY AND ENDOMETRIAL SAMPLING COMPARED WITH D&C

There is evidence that hysteroscopy and directed endometrial biopsy is as good as, and possibly superior to, D&C in the diagnosis of endometrial pathology. A study compared panoramic hysteroscopy and directed biopsy with D&C in over 250 women presenting mainly with abnormal (premenopausal) bleeding.[4] In the majority of women, a similar result was obtained with each procedure; however, in 16% of women, hysteroscopy and biopsy was more revealing than D&C, while

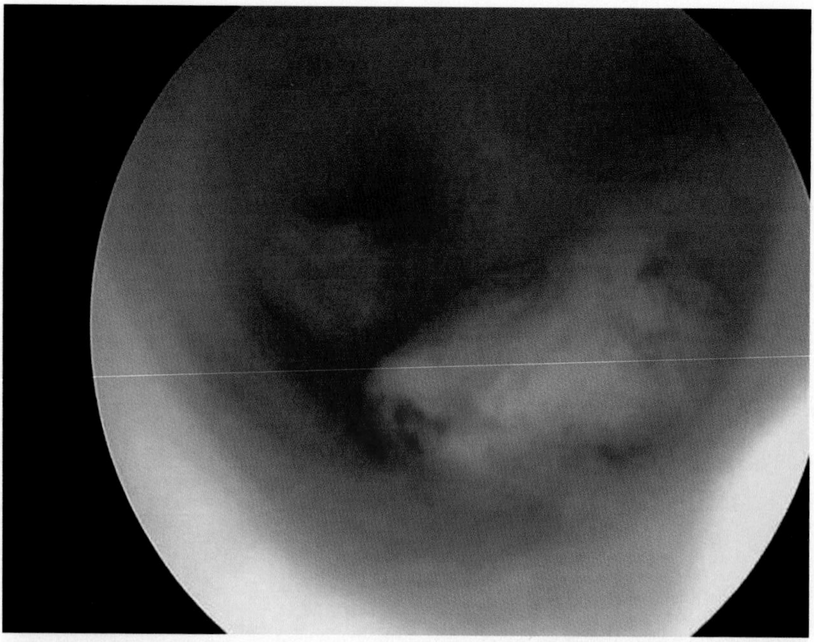

Figure 3.3 Sessile stromal myofibroblast and focal lesion (postmenopausal bleeding)

in only 3% was D&C more revealing. All three cases of endometrial adenocarcinoma were detected with both hysteroscopy and D&C. Another study has shown that endometrial polyps were often missed during conventional D&C but detected by hysteroscopy and biopsy.[5] Two large systematic quantitative reviews have demonstrated good accuracy of hysteroscopy in diagnosing both endometrial and focal pathology.[9,11]

BOX 3.2 KEY POINTS: HYSTEROSCOPY

Hysteroscopy and endometrial sampling:

- should be performed in an outpatient setting with or without local anaesthesia for the majority of women
- is probably more effective than D&C for the detection of endometrial abnormalities
- is the method of choice for diagnosing and treating focal pathologies such as polyps or fibroids associated with abnormal bleeding.

Ultrasound

Ultrasound was introduced for obstetric imaging by Ian Donald working in Glasgow in the 1950s. Its place in routine obstetric and gynaecological practice is now established. In gynaecology, ultrasound is used for the investigation of pelvic masses including fibroids, complications of early pregnancy and assessment of the endometrium.

EQUIPMENT

Structures of different density within the body differ in their ability to transmit ultrasound waves. At the interface between such structures, part of the ultrasound beam is reflected back and can be detected by a sonic sensor and displayed on a screen. The amount of beam reflected is proportional to the difference in density between the tissues. In medicine, frequencies of 1–10 MHz are normally employed. These waves are generated by crystals such as lead zirconate titanate, which convert electrical energy into ultrasound waves. These same crystals can also convert reflected ultrasound waves into an electrical signal, as electrons are released following the compression of the crystal lattice by the returning ultrasound beam. The transducer head containing these crystals acts as both a transmitter and as a sensor for the reflected ultrasound beam. A greyscale picture is computed from the reflected beam. This picture corresponds to a sagittal plane through the body in line with the transducer head. Echodense structures (normally solid organs) appear white, and those organs which allow ultrasound waves to pass with minimal attenuation (such as fluid-filled organs) appear black. In real-time scanning the image is computed many times per second, thus allowing movement of the internal organs to be displayed. Resolution is improved by increasing the frequency of the ultrasound waves; however, this is at the expense of decreased tissue penetration. Maximum tissue penetration is normally limited to 20–70 mm.

Gynaecological ultrasound was initially performed transabdominally using frequencies of 2.5–3.5 MHz. The echotranslucency of a full urinary bladder can be used to push bowel loops out of the pelvis and allow good pictures to be obtained.

Transvaginal ultrasound has become increasingly popular for examination of the ovaries and of the non-pregnant and early pregnant uterus. Transvaginal ultrasound has the advantage that the distance between the end of the ultrasound probe and the pelvic organs is reduced compared with abdominal ultrasound, allowing a higher frequency of ultrasound beam (6–8 MHz) and thus improved resolution. Clearly, however, transvaginal ultrasound is not suitable for women in whom vaginal examination would be avoided. Technological advances in ultrasonic imaging have increased the use of this technique in day-to-day gynaecological practice. These innovations include the miniaturization and portability of equipment, improvements in image quality and three-dimensional imaging.

TECHNIQUE

For all ultrasound examinations a coupling medium of ultrasound gel is used to facilitate transmission of the ultrasound wave from the transducer to the patient. During abdominal ultrasound, the orientation of the ultrasound probe can be used as a guide to the interpretation of ultrasound images. A systematic examination of the pelvic organs is made to assess their structure and contents. During vaginal ultrasound, orientation is more difficult and landmarks such as the iliac vessels may be helpful. Whichever technique is used, it is essential that the operator has had some training in ultrasound so that images are interpreted appropriately.

DIAGNOSIS

Ultrasound can be used to determine the architecture of the uterine body and endometrium. Pelvic ultrasound is more sensitive than vaginal examination in detecting gynaecological disease. Ultrasound is useful in the diagnosis of uterine fibroids as well as for evaluating the ovaries. Operators experienced in gynaecological ultrasound can give an assessment of the nature of the cyst with regard to its morphological appearance (such as size, regularity, septae, presence of echoes suggesting solid areas and so on; see Figure 3.4). Measurement of endometrial thickness by ultrasound is now the first-line test for the investigation of postmenopausal bleeding. The likelihood of endometrial cancer is reduced at endometrial thicknesses below 5 mm. Endometrial biopsy, with or without hysteroscopy, is indicated beyond this threshold.[11–13] Measurements of endometrial thickness vary in women of reproductive age and are less informative because the appearance and thickness of the endometrium change cyclically. However, the regularity, continuity and homogeneity of the endometrium can be assessed for diagnosing focal pathologies such as polyps, submucous fibroids and congenital uterine anomalies. Where focal pathologies are suspected, instillation of saline or gel

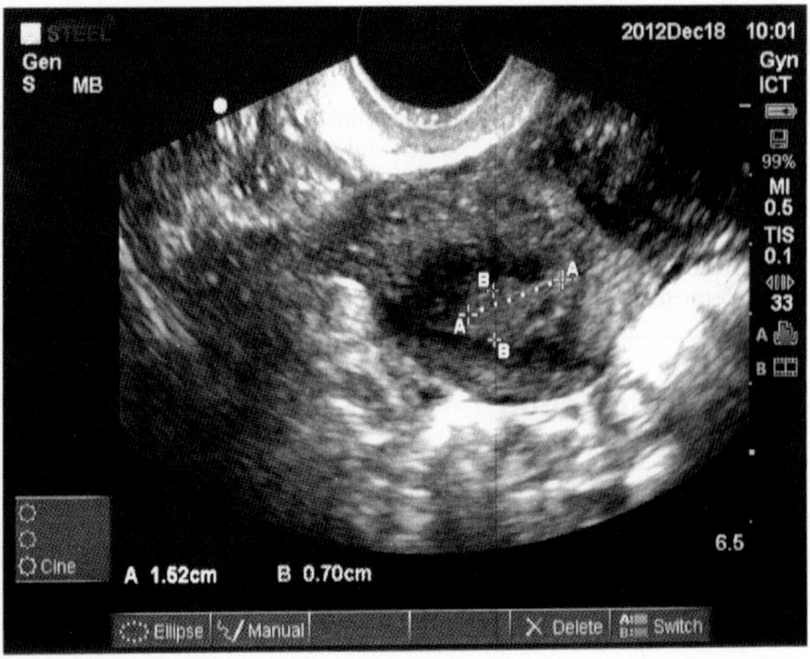

Figure 3.4 Endometrial polyp

through a small catheter placed within the cervix can facilitate diagnosis with a higher level of accuracy.[14,15]

EFFICACY

Measurement of endometrial thickness by transvaginal ultrasound is the recommended first-line test for investigating postmenopausal bleeding. The risk of endometrial cancer is reduced from 5%–10% to under 1% with a negative test (endometrial thickness below 5 mm) such that no further testing is necessary unless symptoms persist. A positive ultrasound necessitates endometrial biopsy with or without recourse to hysteroscopy.[12,16]

SAFETY

To date, there are few data indicating that ultrasound has any adverse effect in non-pregnant women, provided the guidelines for maximum power output are adhered to for each area of the body to be examined.

BOX 3.3 KEY POINTS: ULTRASOUND

Ultrasound:

- is safe and versatile, allowing evaluation of the endometrium, myometrium and ovaries
- can be used to measure endometrial thickness, which should be less than 5 mm in postmenopausal women
- is the most cost-effective first-line test for investigating postmenopausal bleeding for the diagnosis of endometrial carcinoma.

Doppler ultrasound

Doppler ultrasound uses the phenomenon of Doppler shift to measure blood flow through a vessel. Changes in the menstrual cycle and malignant change may be associated with changes in uterine or endometrial blood flow, and therefore can be detected by Doppler ultrasound.

EQUIPMENT

The principle of Doppler ultrasound is that the Doppler shift (the change in frequency of sound waves) coming from a moving target is proportional to the velocity of the target. In medicine, sound waves are generated by an ultrasound transducer. The change in frequency of the reflected wave can be measured by the transducer and the velocity of the target – usually red blood cells – can be determined. If the diameter of the blood vessel and the velocity of the blood cells are known, blood flow can be calculated. However, modern Doppler techniques use waveform analysis to make indirect measurements of flow. This avoids the inevitable errors involved in calculation of blood flow. Many waveform analyses compare systolic (S) and diastolic (D) Doppler frequency shift. The resistance index is (S – D)/S. The pulsatility index is defined as (S – D)/mean. When diastolic flow is high, corresponding to abnormal increased blood flow, the resistance index and pulsatility index are low.

The two main types of Doppler ultrasound are continuous wave and pulsed wave. Continuous wave Doppler employs probes with two crystals, one for receiving and one for transmitting signals. Ultrasound waves are transmitted continuously and the operator relies on pattern recognition of the waveform to identify the correct vessel. The equipment is unable to discriminate between signals coming from different depths. Pulsed wave Doppler uses only one crystal, which operates as both a transmitter and a receiver. The sample volume can be positioned so that only signals coming from a particular distance from the receiver are detected. When pulsed Doppler is combined with real-time ultrasound, the operator can identify the vessel of interest on the screen and display the waveform from that particular vessel. Predictably, pulsed Doppler systems are more expensive and less mobile than continuous wave Doppler; however, they are essential in studies of uterine flow. Colour-flow mapping is a further modification whereby direction and intensity of blood flow within a vessel are indicated by different colours.

TECHNIQUE

Most vessels have a characteristic Doppler waveform which is dependent on both the proximal circulation and the distal receiving bed. Using duplex Doppler (pulsed wave Doppler combined with real-time scanning), the vessel of interest can be identified with B-mode ultrasound and the waveform displayed. As with other ultrasound techniques, a coupling gel is required to improve signal transduction between the end of the probe and the patient.

EFFICACY

Using colour-flow Doppler, flow can be demonstrated in the endometrium in women with endometrial carcinoma. Pelvic tumours, including endometrial tumours, are associated with high diastolic flow and therefore low resistance and pulsatility indices. This finding has been employed to screen for endometrial malignancy in postmenopausal women, including an attempt to improve diagnosis of potential leiomyosarcoma in women with fibroids, since the fibroids themselves are avascular internally but malignancy leads to increased angiogenesis. When abnormality is defined as a pulsatility index of less than 2.00, the sensitivity of this technique to detect endometrial cancer is 99%, with a false-positive rate of only 2.6%.[17] In a study of 750 postmenopausal women scheduled for abdominal hysterectomy, transvaginal colour Doppler ultrasound correctly identified 32 out of 35 women (91.4%) with endometrial carcinoma, using a resistance index of less than 0.4 as a definition of abnormality.[18] The indication for hysterectomy was not stated in this latter study, but none of the women were taking hormone replacement therapy.

These studies suggest that measurements of endometrial blood flow using Doppler techniques may be potentially useful in identifying women with endometrial pathology. However, before this technique can replace histological assessment of the endometrium, more evaluation is required.

BOX 3.4 KEY POINTS: DOPPLER ULTRASOUND

- Doppler ultrasound can be used to measure blood flow.
- Blood flow to the uterus is increased in association with endometrial cancer.
- Further evaluation of this technique is required.

Outpatient endometrial biopsy

Various endometrial samplers have been developed, most based on the Pipelle prototype. These miniature devices have the advantage that the endometrium can be sampled in the clinic at the time of examination without the need for general anaesthesia.

EQUIPMENT

The Pipelle device is a clear, flexible polypropylene cannula approximately 3 mm in diameter. It has a rounded distal tip and a piston inside, which can be withdrawn to create negative pressure. Alternative designs such as the Vabra® aspirator require external suction apparatus so that endometrial samples are drawn into the device.

TECHNIQUE

A speculum (usually Cusco's) is inserted into the vagina so that the cervix can be visualised and a bimanual examination carried out to check the position and size of the uterus, and to feel for adnexal abnormalities. The device is then inserted gently through the cervix into the uterine cavity. If necessary, a volsellum can be applied to the cervix to steady it and to straighten the cervical canal. The exact technique varies according to the device used but the majority are based on the Pipelle design and are manipulated in the following way. The Pipelle cannula is placed at the uterine fundus, the piston is withdrawn to create negative pressure and the device is rotated through 360° and gently withdrawn so that the whole of the endometrial cavity is sampled. The cannula is removed from the uterine cavity and the tissue specimen placed in a specimen pot for histological analysis. This is achieved by either cutting off the top of the Pipelle sampler with scissors or, more commonly, by simply reinserting the piston into the cannula and thereby pushing the collected tissue contained within into the specimen pot. Repeated insertions allow for larger tissue samples.

EFFICACY

Initial concerns over the accuracy of miniature outpatient biopsy in diagnosing serious endometrial pathology arose because of the relatively small area of uterus (4%) found to be sampled by the device.[19] However, most cases of endometrial hyperplasia or cancer affect the endometrium globally and systematic quantitative reviews have shown outpatient endometrial biopsy to have a high overall accuracy in diagnosing endometrial cancer and hyperplasia when adequate specimens are obtained.[20,21] Positive test results were found to be more accurate than negative test results. Therefore, in cases of abnormal uterine bleeding where symptoms persist despite negative biopsy, further evaluation is warranted. In contrast to women of reproductive age with a functional endometrium, non-diagnostic biopsy is not uncommon in postmenopausal women. One in five biopsies fall into this category because of failure to pass the device through a stenosed cervix or because insufficient tissue is obtained from a correctly placed device.[20] In most cases of non-informative biopsy, further diagnostic testing (usually with outpatient hysteroscopy) is indicated, unless the biopsy occurred when the endometrium is very thin.

SAFETY

Uterine perforation is a potential hazard, especially with non-flexible metal devices, particularly if the axis of the uterus is not checked pre-insertion. Miniature plastic Pipelle-type devices are not associated with significant uterine trauma; however, while the procedure is simple and quick and can be integrated into the routine pelvic examination, it can be associated with substantial discomfort.

BOX 3.5 KEY POINTS: OUTPATIENT ENDOMETRIAL BIOPSY

Endometrial samplers:

- can be used to obtain a sample of endometrium for histology
- have high levels of accuracy for diagnosing endometrial cancer.

Indications for uterine cavity evaluation

The gynaecologist is often faced with the situation where a woman in whom history and examination are otherwise normal complains of heavy or irregular periods. The following discussion describes which women require further evaluation in terms of one of the procedures described in this chapter, and which women can be safely treated without further investigation (see also Figure 3.1, page 20).

IS INVESTIGATION REQUIRED TO EXCLUDE ENDOMETRIAL CARCINOMA?

The most pressing reason to evaluate the uterine cavity is to exclude endometrial carcinoma. Clearly, a woman with this condition should have the diagnosis made without delay so that appropriate treatment can be undertaken. The exclusion of endometrial carcinoma is the only reason to evaluate the uterine cavity before a trial of drug therapy. The NICE guidelines emphasise that endometrial adenocarcinoma and pre-malignant adenomatous hyperplasia are uncommon in women under 40 years of age,[22] unless risk factors such as polycystic ovarian syndrome, obesity or tamoxifen use are present. Lewis found that less than 1% of adenocarcinomas of the corpus uteri occurred in women under 35 years of age.[23] The predicted incidence of endometrial adenocarcinoma in women under 35 years of age is less than 1/100 000/year.[24] When hysteroscopy or D&C is performed in young women (under 45 years of age) with heavy menstrual bleeding only, the yield of endometrial carcinoma is negligible.[24,25] These data led to the 2007 NICE recommendation that women with heavy menstrual bleeding only (i.e. regular menstrual cycle) under 45 years of age do not require endometrial biopsy.[22] However, biopsy should be considered in younger women whose symptoms fail to respond to medical treatment, who have persistent inter-menstrual bleeding or who have risk factors for endometrial hyperplasia.

CAN D&C OR HYSTEROSCOPY BE USEFUL IN TREATMENT?

There is clear evidence that D&C does not result in a long-term reduction in menstrual blood loss in women complaining of heavy menstrual bleeding. However, permanent destruction of the basal endometrium using hysteroscopic resection or modern second-generation ablative technologies is very effective in treating this complaint. Evidence suggests that women with abnormal uterine bleeding associated with an endometrial polyp may benefit from its removal.[26] Removal can be effected with blind D&C or avulsion, but such approaches are being superseded by hysteroscopically directed techniques suitable for use in an outpatient setting using bipolar electrosurgery or morcellation[10] (see Chapter 5, Surgical Treatment).

BOX 3.6 KEY POINTS: INDICATIONS FOR UTERINE CAVITY EVALUATION

- The purpose of urgent evaluation is to exclude endometrial carcinoma as a cause of abnormal bleeding.
- Evaluation is not required in women under 45 years of age with a regular menstrual cycle.
- D&C is not useful in the treatment of menstrual disorders.
- All women with postmenopausal bleeding should be investigated urgently by transvaginal ultrasound to measure endometrial thickness.

Conclusion

D&C used to be the established technique for evaluating the uterus in women with menstrual problems. This technique has been largely replaced as a first-line test by more convenient and less invasive pelvic ultrasound, outpatient hysteroscopy and biopsy. Women with refractory menstrual problems, abnormal examination findings or irregular cycles should have prompt endometrial evaluation using these tests. However, the optimal test or combination testing strategy has yet to be determined.[27] Women presenting with postmenopausal bleeding require urgent referral for pelvic ultrasound and further testing, with endometrial biopsy and/or hysteroscopy undertaken depending on the initial ultrasound result.

References

1. Hospital Episode Statistics [www.hesonline.nhs.uk].
2. Monaghan JM (editor). *Rob & Smith's Operative Surgery: Gynaecology and Obstetrics* (4th ed.). London: Butterworths; 1983.
3. Stovall TG, Solomon SK, Ling FW. Endometrial sampling prior to hysterectomy. *Obstet Gynecol* 1989;73:405–8.
4. Gimpleson RJ, Rappold HO. A comparative study between panoramic hysteroscopy with directed biopsies and dilatation and curettage. A review of 276 cases. *Am J Obstet Gynecol* 1988;158:489–92.
5. Loffer FD. Hysteroscopy with selective endometrial sampling compared with D&C for abnormal uterine bleeding: the value of a negative hysteroscopic view. *Obstet Gynecol* 1989;73:16–20.
6. Grimes DA. Diagnostic dilatation and curettage: a reappraisal. *Am J Obstet Gynecol* 1982;142:1–6.
7. Cooper NA, Smith P, Khan KS, Clark TJ. Vaginoscopic approach to outpatient hysteroscopy: a systematic review of the effect on pain. *BJOG* 2010;117:532–9. Erratum in: *BJOG* 2010;117:1440.

8. Royal College of Obstetricians and Gynaecologists, British Society for Gynaecological Endoscopy. *Best Practice in Outpatient Hysteroscopy.* Green-top Guideline no. 59. London: RCOG; 2011 [http://www.rcog.org.uk/womens-health/clinical-guidance/hysteroscopy-best-practice-outpatient-green-top-59].
9. van Dongen H, de Kroon CD, Jacobi CE, Trimbos JB, Jansen FW. Diagnostic hysteroscopy in abnormal uterine bleeding: a systematic review and meta-analysis. *BJOG* 2007;114:664–75.
10. Clark TJ, Gupta JK. *Handbook of Outpatient Hysteroscopy: A Complete Guide to Diagnosis and Therapy*. London: Hodder Arnold; 2005.
11. Clark TJ, Voit D, Gupta JK, Hyde C, Song F, Khan KS. Accuracy of hysteroscopy in the diagnosis of endometrial cancer and disease: a systematic quantitative review. *JAMA* 2002;288:1610–21.
12. Smith-Bindman R, Kerlikowske K, Feldstein VA, et al. Endovaginal ultrasound to exclude endometrial cancer and other endometrial abnormalities. *JAMA* 1998;280:1510–7.
13. Scottish Intercollegiate Guidelines Network. *Investigation of Post-menopausal Bleeding.* A national clinical guideline. Edinburgh: SIGN; 2002 [http://www.sign.ac.uk/guidelines/fulltext/61/index.html].
14. Farquhar C, Ekeroma A, Furness S, Arroll B. A systematic review of transvaginal ultrasonography, sonohysterography and hysteroscopy for the investigation of abnormal uterine bleeding in premenopausal women. *Acta Obstet Gynecol Scand* 2003;82:493–504.
15. de Kroon CD, de Bock GH, Dieben SW, Jansen FW. Saline contrast hysterosonography in abnormal uterine bleeding: a systematic review and meta-analysis. *BJOG* 2003;110:938–47.
16. Clark TJ, Barton PM, Coomarasamy A, Gupta JK, Khan KS. Investigating postmenopausal bleeding for endometrial cancer: cost-effectiveness of initial diagnostic strategies. *BJOG* 2006;113:502–10.
17. Bourne TH, Campbell S, Whitehead MI, Royston P, Steer CV, Collins WP. Detection of endometrial cancer in postmenopausal women by transvaginal ultrasonography and colour flow imaging. *BMJ* 1990;301:369.
18. Kurjak A, Shalan H, Sosic A, et al. Endometrial carcinoma in post menopausal women: evaluation by transvaginal color Doppler ultrasonography. *Am J Obstet Gynecol* 1993;169:1597–603.
19. Rodriguez GC, Yaqub N, King ME. A comparison of the Pipelle device and the Vabra aspirator as measured by endometrial denudation in hysterectomy specimens: the Pipelle device samples significantly less of the endometrial surface than the Vabra aspirator. *Am J Obstet Gynecol* 1993;168:55–9.
20. Clark TJ, Mann CH, Shah N, Khan KS, Song F, Gupta JK. Accuracy of outpatient endometrial biopsy in the diagnosis of endometrial cancer: A systematic quantitative review. *BJOG* 2002;109:313–21.
21. Clark TJ, Mann CH, Shah N, Khan KS, Song F, Gupta JK. Accuracy of outpatient endometrial biopsy in the diagnosis of endometrial hyperplasia. *Acta Obstet Gynecol Scand* 2001;80:784–93.

22. National Institute for Health and Clinical Excellence. *Heavy Menstrual Bleeding*. NICE Clinical Guideline 44. London: NICE; 2007 [http://www.nice.org.uk/guidance/CG44].
23. Lewis BV. Diagnostic dilatation and curettage in young women. *BMJ* 1993;306:225–6.
24. MacKenzie IZ, Bibby JG. Critical assessment of dilatation and curettage in 1029 women. *Lancet* 1978;2:566–8.
25. Fraser IS. Hysteroscopy and laparoscopy in women with menorrhagia. *Am J Obstet Gynecol* 1992;162:1264–9.
26. Nathani F, Clark TJ. Uterine polypectomy in the management of abnormal uterine bleeding: A systematic review. *J Minim Invasive Gynecol* 2006;13:260–8.
27. Critchley HO, Warner P, Lee AJ, Brechin S, Guise J, Graham B. Evaluation of abnormal uterine bleeding: comparison of three outpatient procedures within cohorts defined by age and menopausal status. *Health Technol Assess* 2004;8:1–139.

4 Medical management of excessive menstrual bleeding

Management of excessive menstrual bleeding has changed over the past two decades with the promotion of effective medical treatments and in particular the use of the levonorgestrel-releasing intrauterine device. In the United Kingdom the number of hysterectomies for HMB fell by 36% between 1989 and 2002–3. In NHS hospitals in England in 2006–7, 31 684 abdominal and 6588 vaginal hysterectomies were performed compared with 41 418 and 10 439, respectively, in 1999–2000.[1] Medical management is advocated as initial treatment in women without significant pelvic pathology.[2,3] Medical treatment options and their effectiveness are detailed in Tables 4.1 and 4.2.

The aims of therapy are to reduce blood loss, reduce the risk of anaemia and improve quality of life.[4,5] HMB is the most common cause of iron deficiency anaemia in western women and thus iron therapy is often indicated as well as the options discussed below. It could be

Table 4.1 Medical management of excessive menstrual bleeding

Non-hormonal treatments	*Hormonal treatments*
Non-steroidal anti-inflammatory drugs: • Mefanemic acid • Meclofenamic acid • Naproxen • Ibuprofen • Flurbiprofen • Diclofenac Antifibrinolytics: • Tranexamic acid Other: • Etamsylate	Oral progestogens: • Norethisterone • Medroxyprogesterone acetate • Dydrogetserone Intrauterine progestogens: • Levonorgestrel IUCD • Progestasert IUCD Combined estrogen/progestogens: • Oral contraceptives • Hormone replacement therapy Other: • Danazol • Gestrinone • GnRH analogues • Mifepristone

GnRH = gonadotrophin-releasing hormone agonist; IUCD = intrauterine contraceptive device

Table 4.2 Summary of evidence base for pharmacological interventions in menorrhagia[4]

Treatment	*Reduction of menstrual blood loss*
Nonsteroidal anti-inflammatory drugs	20–49%
Tranexamic acid	29–58%
Etamsylate	About 50% – not clinically significant
Oral progestogens for 21 days	83%
Oral progestogens, luteal administration	Ineffective
*Long-acting progestogen	22–47% of women experience amenorrhoea after 1–2 years of depot medroxyprogesterone acetate use
*Levonorgestrel intrauterine system	71–90%
*Combined oral contraceptive pill	43%
Danazol	About 50%
Gonadotrophin-release hormone agonists	> 90%

* Also provide effective contraception.

argued that menstrual blood loss should be reduced to be within the normal range (less than 80 ml per period). However, women who are keen to avoid surgery may accept a higher loss if they can cope with the flow and any anaemia is controlled with iron supplements.

It is important to assess drug therapies in terms of reduction of measured menstrual blood loss, since there is poor correlation between objective and subjective assessment. Well-designed randomized controlled trials provide the best evidence of the efficacy of any intervention, as any differences between groups can be more confidently attributed to differences in treatment.

Non-hormonal treatment options

NON-STEROIDAL ANTI-INFLAMMATORY DRUGS

Abnormal prostaglandin metabolism has been implicated in excessive menstrual bleeding and thus inhibition of their synthesis with NSAIDs provides an important treatment option.[6] The cyclooxygenase (COX) pathway, with its two main enzyme pathways cyclooxygenase-1 (COX-1) and cyclooxygenase-2 (COX-2), represents one of the major routes for oxidative metabolism of arachidonic acid to prostaglandins. COX inhibitors can be chemically classified into two main groups: COX-1 inhibitors (salicylates [aspirin], indoleacetic acid analogues [indomethacin], aryl propionic acid derivatives [naproxen, ibuprofen] and fenamates [mefenamic acid, flufenamic acid, meclofenamic acid]) and

COX-2 inhibitors (coxibs [celecoxib, rofecoxib]). Studies have been limited to COX-1 inhibitors as uncertainty has been raised regarding the safety of COX-2 inhibitors.

Various COX-1 inhibitors have been evaluated in randomized controlled trials. While reducing menstrual blood loss, the additional benefit of COX-1 inhibitors is that they also improve menstrual pain. In a Cochrane review, five of seven randomized trials showed that mean menstrual blood loss was less with NSAIDs than with placebo, and two showed no difference. Furthermore, there was no evidence that one NSAID (naproxen or mefenamic acid) was superior to the other.[6] The fenamates (such as mefenamic acid) are the most extensively studied NSAIDs. They have the unique property of inhibiting prostaglandin synthesis as well as binding to prostaglandin receptors, whose concentrations are significantly increased in the uteri of women with menorrhagia. The percentage of blood loss reduction varies from 20%–49% depending on the agent and dosage used. A common side effect of NSAIDs is gastrointestinal irritation.

Optimal doses and schedules are difficult to define. Most studies, however, analysed regimens starting on the first day of menstruation and continuing for 5 days or until cessation of menstruation. There does not seem to be an extra advantage in starting therapy before the onset of menstruation which is consistent with the very short half-life (minutes) of prostaglandins.

ANTIFIBRINOLYTICS

Plasminogen activator inhibitors have been promoted as a treatment for excessive menstrual bleeding because of increased endometrial fibrinolytic activity in women with the condition.[7,8] Tranexamic acid taken 2–4.5 g/day for 4 to 7 days reduces menstrual blood flow by 29% to 58% over two to three cycles. The effect is superior to placebo, mefenamic acid, flurbiprofen, etamsylate and oral luteal phase norethisterone at clinically relevant dosages. Side effects are mainly limited to gastrointestinal complaints. Earlier theoretical concerns about thromboembolism caused by antifibrinolytic action of tranexamic acid have not been found in long-term studies.

ETAMSYLATE

Etamsylate is thought to act by reducing capillary fragility, though the precise mechanisms are uncertain. Studies with objective menstrual blood loss measurement using the currently recommended doses show that it is ineffective.[2–4]

Hormonal treatments

PROGESTOGENS

The use of progestogens is based on the erroneous concept that women with excessive menstrual bleeding principally have anovulatory cycles and require progestogen supplementation. Oral, intrauterine and intramuscular depot administration are used.[9–13] The latter are employed mainly for contraception and there is little information regarding menorrhagia.

Intrauterine administration

Intrauterine administration of levonorgestrel (LNG) is very effective. The Mirena® (Bayer, Newbury, Berkshire) intrauterine system (IUS) delivers 20 micrograms of levonorgestrel over 24 hours for about 5 years. Newer, so-called 'frameless' IUS devices are currently being evaluated.[14]

The NICE guideline on HMB published in 2008 recommended the use of Mirena as a first-line agent since it is effective, safe and cost-effective. There are now an increasing number of progestogen-impregnated devices since Mirena is reaching the end of its patent period. These new devices are likely to be smaller and cheaper but there is no reason to believe they will be less effective than the Mirena, which has had a major impact on gynaecological practice. The Progestasert was the first hormonally impregnated device, but prospective randomized studies in HMB are lacking since Progestasert was associated with an increased risk of ectopic pregnancy and was withdrawn from the market. Mirena does not suffer from this adverse effect and has an excellent safety profile.

The Mirena LNG-IUS reduces menstrual blood loss by 71%–90%, and its use has revolutionized management of excessive menstrual bleeding. The LNG-IUS also provides very effective contraception. Its effectiveness has been compared with that of cyclical progestogens, endometrial ablation and hysterectomy. The LNG-IUS is more successful than cyclical norethisterone (for 21 days). Although the LNG-IUS results in a smaller mean reduction in menstrual blood loss (as assessed by pictorial charts) than endometrial ablation, there is no evidence of a difference in the rate of satisfaction with treatment. Women with an LNG-IUS experience more progestogenic adverse effects compared with women having endometrial ablation, although perceived quality of life is similar. This is true also when the LNG-IUS is compared with hysterectomy. However, the LNG-IUS treatment costs less than hysterectomy. One of the few randomized controlled trials using the LNG-IUS for 5 years found a 42% hysterectomy rate, questioning its success in the longer term.[15] The main adverse effect associated with LNG-IUS is frequently occurring variable bleeding and spotting, particularly within the first few months of use. The LNG-IUS is also sometimes associated with the development of ovarian cysts, but these are usually symptomless and show a high rate of spontaneous resolution. It may help with premenstrual symptoms.[16] The LNG-IUS is recommended by the National Institute for Health and Clinical Excellence (NICE) as a first-line treatment, provided long-term use (at least 12 months) is anticipated.[2]

The use of the LNG-IUS for the management of HMB in primary care (as opposed to women recruited to HMB trials with a menstrual blood loss of more than 80 ml, for example objective menorrhagia) is being evaluated.

Oral and intramuscular progestogens

Traditionally, oral progestogen administration was in the luteal phase based on the idea that excessive menstrual bleeding was due to anovulatory cycles. However, studies with measured menstrual blood loss with luteal administration of norethisterone 5 mg twice daily show either a decrease or even an increase in flow.[10] Yet norethisterone 5 mg three times daily from days 5 to 26 of the menstrual cycle is effective, reducing blood loss by 83% in one randomized controlled trial. However, side effects include weight gain, headache and bloatedness, and women find the treatment less acceptable than intrauterine levonorgestrel. There are also concerns that progestogens used in doses greater than those needed in progestogen-only contraception increase the risk of venous thromboembolism.[17]

A systematic review has found that progestogen therapy during the luteal phase was significantly less effective at reducing menstrual blood loss when compared with tranexamic acid, danazol and the LNG-IUS.[10] Duration of menstruation was significantly longer with the LNG-IUS when compared with oral progestogen therapy but significantly shorter with danazol treatment. Adverse events were significantly more likely with danazol when compared with progestogen treatment. Progestogen therapy from days 5 to 26 of the menstrual cycle was significantly less effective at reducing menstrual blood loss than the LNG-IUS. A significantly higher proportion of norethisterone patients taking progestogens found their treatment unacceptable compared with LNG-IUS patients. However, the adverse effects of breast tenderness and inter-menstrual bleeding were more likely in women with the LNG-IUS.

Despite being licensed as a contraceptive, Depo-Provera® (Pfizer Inc, USA), an intramuscular medroxyprogesterone acetate, is often used to treat HMB as it can induce amenorrhoea. However, there are no randomized controlled trial data. There are also no data concerning progestogen-only pills or subdermal implants.

Oestrogen/progestogen combinations

From clinical experience, combined oral contraceptives (COCs) are generally considered to be effective in the management of dysfunctional menstrual bleeding. However, there are few available data to support this observation with the 20–35 microgram ethinylestradiol-containing pills in current practice.[18,19] Studies are mainly limited to higher dose COCs. There are no data with the contraceptive patch. Alternative regimens to be considered are inducing bleeds every 3 months or taking the COC without a break; however, neither regimen has been studied in menorrhagia.

With regard to sequential oestrogen/progestogen hormone replacement therapy regimens, although the induced withdrawal bleeds are not excessive there have been no trials in menorrhagia.

Others

Danazol is an isoxazol derivative of 17 alpha-ethinyl-testosterone which acts on the hypothalamic–pituitary axis as well as on the endometrium to produce atrophy. Danazol reduces menstrual blood loss by about 50%.[20] It appears to be more effective than placebo, progestogens, NSAIDs and COCs at reducing menstrual loss. Treatment with danazol causes more adverse events than NSAIDs and progestogens. While an effective therapy, its clinical use is limited by androgenic side effects, which are experienced by up to three-quarters of patients. In addition, women must be advised to use barrier methods of contraception because of potential virilization of a fetus if pregnancy occurs while on danazol treatment. It is now rarely used in clinical practice.

Gestrinone is a 19-nortestosterone derivative which has antiprogestogenic, anti-estrogenic and androgenic activity. In a placebo-controlled study it reduced menstrual blood loss in 79% of patients with objective menorrhagia.[5] However it also has androgenic side effects, which limit its long-term use and again women must be advised to use barrier methods of contraception because of potential virilization of a fetus.

Gonadotrophin-releasing hormone (GnRH) agonists, administered continuously or in depot form, down-regulate expression of GnRH receptors, which blocks gonadotrophin secretion from the anterior pituitary. This leads to ovarian suppression. GnRH agonists have been mainly used in fibroid-associated bleeding. Concerns about the long-term effects of ovarian suppression such as osteoporosis generally limit use beyond six months, even when add-back therapy (estrogen/progestogen hormone replacement therapy) is used in conjunction.[5]

Antiprogestogens

Progestogen receptor modulators are discussed in more detail in Chapter 6. Mifepristone (RU-486) is a synthetic 19-norsteroid with antiprogestogen activity that has been shown to inhibit ovulation and to disrupt endometrial integrity.[21] Mifepristone was recently shown to act as a contraceptive agent and to induce amenorrhea at a dosage of 5 mg per day in the majority of women studied. However, there are concerns that it induces endometrial hyperplasia and further research is required.[22]

Asoprisnil, an orally active selective progesterone receptor modulator, was studied for the management of symptomatic uterine leiomyomata as well as HMB with no pathology. Menstrual bleeding was reduced.[23] However, this drug is not being further developed owing to the potential for endometrial pathology to develop.

Ulipristal has recently been licensed for short-term use in the UK. It is extremely effective in reducing menstrual blood loss and is very well tolerated, but it leads to unusual endometrial histology and further evaluation is required before the licence is extended.[24,25]

Patient information, decision aids and choice

It is essential to give the patient information about management options so that she can make an informed choice. The importance of information and counselling was illustrated in a randomized controlled trial of 900 women.[26] Women were randomized to the control group, information alone group (information), or information plus interview group (interview). Hysterectomy rates were lower for women in the interview group than in the control group (48%) and women who received the information alone (48%). NICE also produces information for patients following the development of all guidelines.

Conclusion

Management of excessive menstrual bleeding will depend significantly on the patient's contraceptive needs. NICE recommends the LNG-IUS as the first-line option in women requiring contraception although obviously, it is not suitable for women who wish to conceive in the short term. There is currently no evidence that alternative and complementary therapies reduce menstrual blood loss.

References

1. Hospital episode statistics (HES) online. Main procedures and interventions: 3 character [http://www.hesonline.nhs.uk/Ease/servlet/ContentServer?siteID=1937&categoryID=205].
2. National Institute for Health and Clinical Excellence. *Heavy Menstrual Bleeding: Investigation and Treatment.* Clinical guideline 44. London; NICE: 2007 [http://www.nice.org.uk/guidance/CG44].
3. Oehler MK, Rees MC. Menorrhagia: an update. *Acta Obstet Gynecol Scand* 2003;82:405–22.
4. NHS Evidence. *Clinical Knowledge Summaries: Menorrhagia* [http://www.cks.library.nhs.uk/menorrhagia].
5. Map of Medicine Heavy Menstrual Bleeding (HMB) – primary care [http://healthguides.mapofmedicine.com/choices/map/menstrual_cycle_irregularities_and_post_menopausal_bleeding_pmb_3.html]
6. Lethaby A, Augood C, Duckitt K, Farquhar C. Nonsteroidal anti-inflammatory drugs for heavy menstrual bleeding. *Cochrane Database Syst Rev* 2007;(4):CD000400.
7. Lethaby A, Farquhar C, Cooke I. Antifibrinolytics for heavy menstrual bleeding. *Cochrane Database Syst Rev* 2007;CD000249.
8. Naoulou B, Tsai MC. Efficacy of tranexamic acid in the treatment of idiopathic and non-functional heavy menstrual bleeding: A systematic review. *Acta Obstet Gynecol Scand*. 2012 Jan 10. doi: 10.1111/j.1600–0412.2012.01361.x. [Epub ahead of print].
9. Lethaby AE, Cooke I, Rees M. Progesterone or progestogen-releasing intrauterine systems for heavy menstrual bleeding. *Cochrane Database Syst Rev* 2005;(4):CD002126.
10. Lethaby A, Irvine G, Cameron I. Cyclical progestogens for heavy menstrual bleeding. *Cochrane Database Syst Rev* 2008;(1):CD001016.
11. Roberts TE, Tsourapas A, Middleton LJ. Hysterectomy, endometrial ablation, and levonorgestrel releasing intrauterine system (Mirena) for treatment of heavy menstrual bleeding: cost effectiveness analysis. *BMJ* 2011;342:d2202.
12. Bhattacharya S, Middleton LJ, Tsourapas A, et al.; International Heavy Menstrual Bleeding Individual Patient Data Meta-analysis Collaborative Group. Hysterectomy, endometrial ablation and Mirena® for heavy menstrual bleeding: a systematic review of clinical effectiveness and cost-effectiveness analysis. *Health Technol Assess* 2011;15:iii–xvi, 1–252.
13. Kaunitz AM, Meredith S, Inki P, Kubba A, Sanchez-Ramos L. Levonorgestrel-releasing intrauterine system and endometrial ablation in heavy menstrual bleeding: a systematic review and meta-analysis. *Obstet Gynecol* 2009;113:1104–16.

14. Wildemeersch D. Intrauterine drug delivery for contraception and gynaecological treatment: novel approaches. *Handb Exp Pharmacol* 2010;197:267–98.
15. Hurskainen R, Teperi J, Rissanen P, et al. Clinical outcomes and costs with the levonorgestrel-releasing intrauterine system or hysterectomy for treatment of menorrhagia: randomized trial 5-year follow-up. *JAMA* 2004;291:1456–63.
16. Leminen H, Heliövaara-Peippo S, Halmesmäki K, et al. The effect of hysterectomy or levonorgestrel-releasing intrauterine system on premenstrual symptoms in women treated for menorrhagia: secondary analysis of a randomised controlled trial. *Acta Obstet Gynecol Scand* 2012;91:279–400.
17. Vasilakis C, Jick H, del Mar Melero-Montes M. Risk of idiopathic venous thromboembolism in users of progestogens alone. *Lancet* 1999;354:1610–11.
18. Maguire K, Westhoff C. The state of hormonal contraception today: established and emerging noncontraceptive health benefits. *Am J Obstet Gynecol* 2011;205(4 Suppl):S4–8.
19. Micks E, Jensen JT. Estradiol valerate and dienogest: a novel four-phasic oral contraceptive pill effective for pregnancy prevention and treatment of heavy menstrual bleeding. *Womens Health (Lond Engl)* 2011;7:513–24.
20. Beaumont H, Augood C, Duckitt K, Lethaby A. Danazol for heavy menstrual bleeding. *Cochrane Database Syst Rev* 2007;(3):CD001017.
21. Brown A, Cheng L, Lin S, Baird DT. Daily low-dose mifepristone has contraceptive potential by suppressing ovulation and menstruation: a double-blind randomized control trial of 2 and 5 mg per day for 120 days. *J Clin Endocrinol Metab* 2002;87:63–70.
22. Eisinger SH, Bonfiglio T, Fiscella K, Meldrum S, Guzick DS. Twelve-month safety and efficacy of low-dose mifepristone for uterine myomas. *J Minim Invasive Gynecol* 2005;12:227–33.
23. Wilkens J, Chwalisz K, Han C, et al. Effects of the selective progesterone receptor modulator asoprisnil on uterine artery blood flow, ovarian activity, and clinical symptoms in patients with uterine leiomyomata scheduled for hysterectomy. *J Clin Endocrinol Metab* 2008;93:4664–71.
24. Donnez J, Tatarchuk TF, Bouchard P, et al.; PEARL I Study Group. Ulipristal acetate versus placebo for fibroid treatment before surgery. *N Engl J Med* 2012;366:409–20.
25. Donnez J, Tomaszewski J, Vázquez F, et al.; PEARL II Study Group. Ulipristal acetate versus leuprolide acetate for uterine fibroids. *N Engl J Med* 2012;366:421–32.
26. Kennedy AD, Sculpher MJ, Coulter A, Dwyer N, Rees M, Abrams KR, et al. Effects of decision aids for menorrhagia on treatment choices, health outcomes, and costs: a randomized controlled trial. *JAMA* 2002;288: 2701–8.

5 Surgical management of menstrual problems

While effective medical treatments exist, many women will still ultimately require surgical treatment. This is either through preference, a dislike of medical treatments or the failure or unsuitability of medical treatments.

The surgical options for the management of menstrual problems are chiefly endometrial ablation as a uterine conserving procedure and either total or subtotal hysterectomy, which can be performed by a number of routes. Myomectomy as a fertility-preserving surgical treatment for fibroids confers a menstrual benefit and is discussed in Chapter 6.

Since the first edition of this text was published, several key publications have expanded the knowledge and evidence base of surgical treatment. These are:

- the MISTLETOE Study[1] and the Scottish National Hysteroscopy Audit[2] – two national audits of first-generation endometrial ablation techniques
- the eVALuate study – a randomized controlled trial comparing laparoscopic, abdominal and vaginal hysterectomy[3]
- the VALUE national hysterectomy study – a randomized controlled trial comparing vaginal and abdominal hysterectomy[4]
- NICE Guideline on Heavy Menstrual Bleeding – a national evidence-based guideline on the management of menstrual disorders[5]
- Cochrane reviews of medical versus surgical management of HMB[6] and endometrial ablation versus hysterectomy[7]
- a review and analysis of hysterectomy, endometrial destruction and the LNG-IUS for HMB.[8]

Current methods are discussed below.

Endometrial ablation

Endometrial ablation represents the most thoroughly evaluated surgical treatment to date. Endometrial ablative techniques were first introduced in the 1980s by Goldrath's[9] work on endometrial laser ablation

(ELA) in the US and Magos's[10] work on transcervical resection of the endometrium (TCRE) in the UK. All endometrial ablative techniques aim to create a therapeutic Asherman's syndrome by destroying the basal endometrium resulting in either normal periods (eumenorrhea), light periods (hypomenorrhoea) or complete absence of periods (amenorrhoea). Compared to hysterectomy endometrial ablation offers shorter operating times, rapid recovery, day case procedures and less morbidity.[7]

PATIENT SELECTION FOR ABLATION/OUTCOMES

Ablative procedures should only be offered to a woman whose family is complete. Reliable methods of contraception are required as ablative procedures in themselves do not prevent pregnancy and when this does occur, the outcome is usually poor.

For all ablative techniques that do not provide a pathology specimen the endometrium should be assessed histologically to exclude malignant and premalignant lesions. Previous classical section/myomectomy/hysterotomy are contraindications for second-generation techniques. Active pelvic infection is a contraindication. Cavity sizes should be measured preoperatively as cavities greater than 12 cm have poor outcomes. Optimal outcomes are seen in small regular cavities (10 cm or less). Extreme care should be exercised with immobile uteri (such as fixed retroverted uteri) as they are at a higher risk of difficult dilation and uterine wall damage; ideally, only techniques utilizing direct vision during active treatment should be used in this instance, if at all. Patients should be counselled regarding expected outcomes quoting established data. Normal or light periods should be the expected outcome. Amenorrhea is not guaranteed but should be seen as a bonus. Women should be given written information regarding their procedure and counselled about relative risks. They should be willing to accept the risk of laparoscopy, laparotomy and/or hysterectomy should complication arise. Certain ablative techniques are unsuitable for irregular or fibroid cavities. Certain other prognostic factors exist. Women whose menstrual blood loss is genuinely excessive have a better outcome after ablation than those with normal loss.[11] Patient age may be important as younger women have lower reported satisfaction than older women. The Scottish Audit of Hysteroscopic Surgery showed a lower satisfaction in women under 40 years of age, though this was still 79% as compared to 88% in women aged over 40.[2] The presence of irregular periods or menstrual dysmenorrhoea is not a predictor of a poor outcome.[12] Menstrual dysmenorrhoea is reduced significantly

Table 5.1 First- and second-generation endometrial ablation techniques

First-generation	*Second-generation*
• Transcervical resection of the endometrium • Rollerball endometrial ablation • Endometrial laser ablation	• Thermal balloon ablation • Microwave endometrial ablation (MEA®) • NovaSure® (Hologic, Inc., Bedford, MA, USA) • Hydro ThermAblator® (Boston Scientific, Natick, MA, USA) • Cryosurgical ablation

postablation whereas premenstrual dysmenorrhoea (pain before the bleeding starts) responds poorly.[12,13]

Box 5.1 lists favourable prognostic indicators for endometrial ablation.

BOX 5.1 FAVOURABLE PROGNOSTIC INDICATORS FOR ENDOMETRIAL ABLATION

- Genuine heavy menstrual bleeding (> 80 ml)
- Regular cavity
- Cavity 10 cm or less

Endometrial techniques are divided into first-generation and second-generation techniques (Table 5.1).

FIRST-GENERATION TECHNIQUES

These techniques include TCRE, rollerball endometrial ablation (RBEA) and ELA. These techniques are performed under general anaesthesia. They offer the benefit of direct vision and require a fluid distension media. GnRH analogues are often used to pharmacologically prepare (thin) the endometrium prior to first-generation techniques. GnRH analogues improve vision, improve clinical effect and reduce intra-operative fluid absorption, but with an increased health service cost and a greater risk of difficulty in cervical dilatation.[14]

TCRE was initially performed with modified urological resectoscopes. The technique utilises monopolar electrosurgery which passes a current through a 3 mm 90° cutting loop. This technique usually involves a combination of rollerball ablation to the thinner cornual and difficult to resect fundal regions and resection to the remainder of the endometrial cavity. The 3 mm cutting loop destroys tissue to a total depth of 5 mm with resection of 3 mm of tissue and a zone of thermal necrosis extending a further 2 mm. A pathology specimen is produced by the operation.

As monopolar electrical energy is used the uterine distension media is required to be non-ionic. The most common media in the UK is 1.5% glycine as used by the urologists. This allows conduction of electricity, is non miscible with blood (improving vision) and doesn't form carbon deposits. A complication of its use is a condition first seen in urology – the post-transurethral resection of the prostate syndrome or post-TURP syndrome. This is a serious and occasionally fatal complication. If glycine is absorbed through uterine vessels or transperitoneally, the potential to cause significant hyponatraemia or hyperammonaemia is present. Cerebral oedema (confusion, agitation, fits, coma), pulmonary oedema and metabolic acidosis can occur. Cases of death from respiratory arrest with compression of the respiratory centres due to cerebral tonsillar herniation have been reported.[15,16] Current recommendations limit total fluid absorption to a maximum of 1500 ml, with the advice to abandon the procedure if this limit is approached. A two-stage procedure with a re-operation at a later date is safer. Other complications include uterine perforation, false passage formation, cervical laceration, vascular injury, visceral injury including bowel injury, endometritis and emergency hysterectomy. Antibiotic prophylaxis such as co-amoxiclav 1.2 g intravenously at induction is an option (non-evidence based) used by many experts in the field as transient bacteraemia is common (1%)[17] and rare cases of fatal septicaemia have been reported.[18] TCRE has been compared in a number of randomized controlled trials against hysterectomy and is seen as the gold standard ablative technique to which all others are compared.[11,19–21] In these randomized controlled trials the effectiveness of TCRE was demonstrated giving high levels of satisfaction that was similar to but always less than hysterectomy. Low re-operation rates are reported with only 20%–25% progressing over time to hysterectomy. Most occur in the first 3 years post-ablation.[22] A recent development with resection is newer bipolar resectoscopes which utilise normal saline as a distension media, avoiding the risks of glycine.

RBEA is a similar technique to TCRE except a rolling ball electrode is used to apply monopolar energy to ablate the endometrium. Glycine is required and endometrial preparation recommended. This is the commonest first-generation technique in the USA.

ELA is the least common technique probably because of the significant expenditure required for a laser machine. It utilizes neodymium-YAG laser energy in normal saline as a distension media and pharmacological preparation is recommended.

Safety of first-generation techniques

The incidence of complications following the hysteroscopic methods of TCRE and ELA has been determined by the Scottish Audit of Hysteroscopic Surgery[2] and by the MISTLETOE study in England and Wales,[1] between them giving the results from over 11 000 patients. In both audits it was estimated that over 90% of procedures were reported and that there was no difference in the complication rate in the unreported group. In the MISTLETOE study of over 10 000 cases the rate of bowel damage due to TCRE was 0.7/1000.[1] The Scottish Audit of Hysteroscopy Surgery of just under 1000 cases reported no incidence of bowel damage. RBEA is a first-generation method derived from TCRE and felt to be a safer method as the surface of the uterine cavity is coagulated rather than resected. No visceral damage was reported with this method in MISTLETOE, but there were only 650 cases.[1] There have been a number of case reports of large and small bowel damage after RBEA.[23,24] In the MISTLETOE study the rate of emergency hysterectomy was 6/1000 overall, but 11/1000 when TCRE was performed using a loop for the whole procedure. In the Scottish audit the emergency hysterectomy rate was 2/1000, considerably lower than the English audit. Uterine perforation is reported in 15/1000 cases in the MISTLETOE and 10/1000 in the Scottish Audit.[1,2] This is of little consequence if the perforation is recognized and does not involve the use of electrodiathermy or laser energy.

In MISTLETOE there was a 1% rate of fluid absorption of greater than 2000 ml and 1% in the Scottish Audit. Both audits and a randomized controlled trial comparing TCRE to ELA have shown a greater rate of fluid absorption following ELA as compared to TCRE.[1,2,25] However, as saline is used with ELA, the increased fluid absorption post-ELA is not as much of a concern as it is with TCRE. Combining the two audit studies the mortality from the hysteroscopic methods of endometrial resection and ablation was 0.27/1000.[1,2] In conclusion, the two studies reported on over 11 000 cases and ELA and RBEA were revealed as the safest techniques (although with a lower number of procedures performed), with higher rates of perforation and emergency hysterectomy seen in the TCRE cases.

Post-tubal sterilisation syndrome[26–28] is a late complication associated with endometrial ablations. It occurs when cervical stenosis prevents menstrual loss draining transcervically and tubal sterilization prevents retrograde menstruation. The resulting haematometra causes dilation of the proximal portion of the fallopian tube, resulting in a history of post-ablation cyclical pelvic pain, occasionally an adnexal mass, raised CA125 and tenderness. Many mimic ovarian pathologies such as ovarian cancer or cyst accidents.[29,30]

Pregnancies have been reported following ablation. Many advise offering women sterilization as a permanent method of contraception at the time of ablation if they are not already sterilised or utilizing reliable contraception. The concerns over the safety of the mother and the pregnancy are significant. The risks are miscarriage, preterm labour, intrauterine growth retardation, placental implantation abnormalities (placenta accreta, increta, percreta) and abruption. Occasional normal outcomes have been recorded, but such are the concerns over the risks to the mother and unborn child that therapeutic abortion is to be recommended. Up to June 2002, Cook et al.[31] reviewed the reported pregnancies post ablation. They reported only 17 pregnancies progressing beyond 20 weeks and a single successful term pregnancy.

SECOND-GENERATION TECHNIQUES

First-generation endometrial ablative techniques are difficult procedures to master with long learning curves. Often they are used only where fibroid resection is also being undertaken. Second-generation ablative techniques evolved to simplify the technique and ideally place endometrial ablation safely in the hands of all gynaecologists. The majority use tissue heating as the method of endometrial destruction, using electrical energy (NovaSure® System; Hologic UK Ltd, Crawley, Sussex – bipolar mesh), microwave energy (microwave endometrial ablation or MEA®; Microsulis Medical Ltd, Hampshire, UK), laser (endometrial laser intrauterine thermotherapy [ELITT™]), heated saline/glycine irrigating the uterus (Hydro ThermAblator®; Boston Scientific, Natick, USA]) or heated saline/dextrose contained within a balloon device (Gynecare Thermachoice®; Ethicon Women's Health and Urology UK, Livingston, Edinburgh and Cavaterm™ systems; Pnn Medical, Morges, Switzerland). Second-generation techniques with the exception of Hydro ThermAblator are blind in nature (no hysteroscopy), and most avoid the need for fluid distension media and its risks. They are quicker and much simpler to learn and perform than first-generation techniques, which many gynaecologists found difficult or impossible to master. Some also offer the benefits of local anaesthesia/outpatient procedures (MEA and Gynecare Thermachoice®).[32,33]

These new procedures all postdate the earlier national safety audits.[1,2] Their efficacy should be compared in randomized trials of adequate power to the now-established gold standard of TCRE. Adequate training is vital to reduce the potential for serious complications with the second-generation techniques. While many techniques do not insist on hysteroscopy, many experts have always recommended that a postdilatation hysteroscopy be performed prior to all blind second-generation techniques to exclude perforation, false passage or uterine wall trauma.

The methods which have been subject to adequate assessment to date are Gynecare Thermachoice,[2,34–36] MEA,[37,38] the Vesta system (Valleylab, Colorado, USA),[39] NovaSure device,[40] Her Option™ (CryoGen Inc., San Diego, USA)[41] and the Hydro ThermAblator.[42]

There have been concerns raised by the Medicines and Healthcare Products Regulatory Agency regarding significant serious complications when second-generation devices have caused extrauterine burns – for example bowel or bladder injury. Postdilatation, preprocedure hysteroscopy and/or intraoperative ultrasound are recommended.[43] The US Food and Drug Administration (FDA) has the MAUDE database recording all complications for second-generation ablative techniques, which can be accessed through the FDA website.[44]

Thermal balloon ablation

Two techniques exist (both approved by NICE): Gynecare Thermachoice® and Cavaterm™. These techniques require a regular cavity. The thermachoice thermal balloon utilizes a catheter that is 16 cm long and 3.1 mm in diameter. Three cables link the device to the control unit. One is the electrical connection, the second the fluid line and the third supplies the impeller. The distensible silicone balloon is filled with 5% dextrose solution at a working temperature of 87 °C and a distending wall pressure of 160–180 mmHg. Treatments are completed in 8 minutes. A predictable 5 mm endometrial thermal destruction is achieved when utilizing these parameters.

Gynecare Thermachoice® III, the currently marketed version, contains an impeller which circulates the dextrose solution to ensure a uniform thermal effect (previous models were troubled by uneven heating). The technique is blind and after sounding of the cavity dilatation is rarely required. The device requires a minimum of 150 mmHg pressure before the heating element is activated. Failure to maintain this pressure will result in an automatic cut-off if pressures exceed 200 mmHg or less than 45 mmHg. Prior to treatment the catheter requires priming with 5% dextrose to establish the balloon is intact and it is then inserted into the cavity and filled with between 10 and 30 ml of dextrose to stabilise the pressure at 160–180 mmHg. Extra dextrose can be introduced during treatment if a small pressure fall (as a result of uterine relaxation) is encountered, a larger drop however should raise concerns of a leaking balloon or a uterine wall defect. Randomized controlled trial evidence versus RBEA with 5-year follow-up revealed amenorrhoea rates of 15% and satisfaction rates of 75%. The ability to perform the procedure as an outpatient procedure has been assessed in methodologically sound trials.[33]

Cavaterm™ – a thermal balloon endometrial ablation device – is similar to Gynecare Thermachoice® in that it utilizes a silicone balloon filled with heated dextrose solution. Similarly, it uses an impeller to circulate the heated solution and takes 10 minutes to complete therapy. The main difference is that the Cavaterm™ balloon has an adjustable balloon length to allow treatment of cavities from 5 to 10 cm in depth. Cavaterm™ has been compared to the gold standard of TCRE[45] for the treatment of menorrhagia and should be considered an effective therapeutic option.

Microwave endometrial ablation (MEA)

MEA is approved by NICE. It uses an 8 mm diameter probe that delivers microwaves of a set frequency of 9.2GHz. The microwave frequency and wavelength utilized in MEA® was specifically chosen so that the total depth of thermal effect matched the endometrial thickness, but did not exceed total wall thickness. The selected microwaves result in a predictable 3mm depth of direct microwave penetration and a further 2mm depth of thermal transmission. Thus in total a reliable 5 mm depth of penetration can be achieved. The microwaves radiate from the tip of the probe in a hemispherical array. The probe itself consists of an aluminium tube, which delivers through a ceramic dielectric wave guide the microwave energy that is generated in the magnetron (microwave generator). The energy is radiated in a dielectric hemisphere at the tip of the probe. The probe has two thermocouples, one at the tip to measure the temperature at the tissue surface and another 10 cm down the shaft of the probe to measure any reflected energy and ensure the shaft does not overheat. The temperature at the tip of the probe is relayed to the microwave unit and displayed as a continuous visual temperature display. This allows the operator to guide treatment of the cavity and maintain the temperature within the therapeutic range of 70–80 °C that results in endometrial and superficial myometrial cell death. The continuous temperature monitoring also serves as a safety feature in that if temperatures of above 85 °C occur an audible alarm will sound and the generator will automatically shut off once the temperature reaches 90 °C.

The probe itself is a reusable single piece device that is 338 mm long and 8.5 mm in diameter at the shaft. The probe is covered in a polymer: fluorinated ethylene propylene. The shaft is marked with graduations in whole centimetres. For a distance of 35 mm from the tip a black band extends to indicate the endocervical canal. A yellow band extends for 7 mm below the black band and indicates that the tip of the probe is imminent to prevent haematometra formation that can arise from inadvertently treating the endocervical canal. The MEA® applicator is attached to the system by two cables. The first is the coaxial cable that carries the microwave energy from the microwave generator to the MEA® probe. The second is a data cable that relays continuous information from the thermocouples to the console display and communicates with the chip inside the applicator that stores treatment data and records the number of treatments (set at a maximum of 30).

In a randomized controlled trial MEA® has been compared to TCRE with data extending up to 5 years.[46] MEA has also been compared against Gynecare Thermachoice® in a randomized controlled trial.[47] Cavities up to 12 cm can be treated including cavities with up to 3 cm non-obstructing fibroids/polyps. Previous lower segment caesarean sections require an ultrasound measurement of the lower scar thickness in the anteroposterior dimension of 10 mm or greater prior to MEA®. It has randomized controlled trial evidence of the acceptability and satisfaction of the treatment under local anesthesia. Amenorrhoea rates of up to 65% have been reported at 1 year.

Hysteroscopy after dilatation of the cervix is recommended to ensure that no unintended perforation has occurred.

Please note that in 2011 Microsulis, the manufacturer of MEA, was bought out by Hologic, and MEA is in the process of being phased out of the UK market. However, it is still available outside the UK.

NovaSure®

NovaSure® is a second-generation device that uses a conformable, three-dimensional bipolar gold-plated mesh mounted on an expandable frame to deliver bipolar energy to the cavity.[48] The procedure is performed under general anaesthesia. The device has a disposable handheld instrument 7.2 mm in diameter that is suitable for cavities of between 4 cm and 12 cm in length. Energy delivery is regulated by two factors: firstly the cavity length and width measurements that are input to the control unit by the operator; secondly by the measurement of tissue impedance. The progressive vaporization and desiccation of the tissues caused by the electrical energy increases tissue impedance as tissue water content diminishes. The endometrium is vaporized and evacuated by the constant suction applied to the cavity during the procedure. The myometrium desiccates and once the tissue impedance reaches 50 Ohms the device automatically terminates the procedure. This tissue impedance factor allows the device to be used on unprepared uteri and even during active menstruation by regulating energy delivery, only terminating treatment once the tissue impedance reaches the set 50 Ohms that represents adequate treatment. Average active treatment time is 90 seconds, representing the fastest second-generation technique. Prior to activation the device has a cavity integrity assessment feature utilizing carbon dioxide to insufflate the cavity to a set pressure (50 mmHg) which must be maintained for 4 seconds. Neither preoperative pharmacological preparation nor immediate preoperative hysteroscopy are required.

The NovaSure® device has been compared in a randomized controlled trial to hysteroscopic wire loop resection plus rollerball with follow-up to one year.[40] Amenorrhoea rates of between 41% and 59% have been reported in series.

Hydro ThermAblator®

Unlike the rest of the second-generation techniques, the Hydro ThermAblator® requires hysteroscopy and gives a view of the cavity during active treatment. No manipulation of the device is required once it is placed in the uterine cavity. The technique relies upon circulating heated saline within the endometrial cavity. The saline is heated externally prior to being introduced into the hysteroscope and achieves an intrauterine temperature of 90 °C. The fluid is constantly recirculated at a rate of 300 ml/min. This method is suitable for cavity lengths from 4 cm and for irregular and fibroid cavities, unlike the balloon methods. Intrauterine temperature can be maintained with cavities up to a volume of 60 ml, although this size of cavity is unlikely to be selected for ablation (10–30 ml is the average). The device is 7.8 mm in diameter and takes 10 minutes of active treatment, with a post-treatment cool-down of 1 minute prior to device removal. A pretreatment test run using saline at room temperature is carried out to ensure the circuit is intact; a loss of only 10 ml from the system will trigger an automatic shutdown. The intrauterine pressure is maintained at a net pressure of 50–55 mmHg, thus preventing spillage from the fallopian tubes, which is only apparent at 70 mmHg or above.[49,50] An adequate seal at the cervix is imperative and care must be taken not to over-dilate the cervix. The pressure is maintained by the balance between the hydrostatic mechanism and the pump evacuating the saline from the cavity. The saline is suspended from a dedicated intravenous pole 115 cm above the patient's uterus. The main advantages of the technique are the preoperative hysteroscopic view of the cavity (to exclude false passage/perforation formation) with saline at room temperature; the fact that the device can accommodate any hysteroscope up to 3 mm or smaller;

and the ability of the technique to treat irregular cavities. However, a pharmacological endometrial preparation is essential, which is expensive, causes side effects and increases cervical resistance.

The ability to perform the procedure under local anaesthesia is reported. Amenorrhoea rates of 40% at 1 year are also reported.

Cryosurgical techniques

Her Option® is the endometrial ablative technique that uses cryosurgical endometrial ablation to produce the desired effect on the endometrium and myometrium. The device uses a mixed gas coolant to generate temperatures of –90 °C to –100 °C. Irreversible tissue death is seen at temperatures below –20 °C. The device utilises a 5.5 mm probe that incorporates an electric heater, a thermocouple and a saline flush port. Intraoperative ultrasound is required. Treatment is monitored with ultrasound that reveals the extent of ice ball formation and by the thermocouple display. The leading edge of the ice front corresponds to –1 °C to –2 °C and the ultrasound image corresponds to within 1 mm of the actual depth of the cryo-lesion.[51] Instillation of 300–400 ml of warm saline into the bladder facilitates ultrasound scanning. The probe is inserted into the cavity, its fundal position confirmed by ultrasound, and 5 ml of saline is instilled into the cavity to couple the probe to the endometrial tissues. Treatment begins with the probe angled to the first cornua to be treated. On average three ice balls are required, with the probe tip thawed (via the electric heater) to allow disengagement and repositioning of the device.

A randomized controlled trial of Her Option® cryoablation versus rollerball ablation has been reported.[52] Success, defined as a Pictorial Bleeding Assessment Chart score less than 75 (corresponding to eumenorrhoea), was seen in 77.3% after cryoablation and 83.8% after rollerball ablation. Ninety-two per cent of cryoablations were performed under local anaesthesia. The use of a freezing effect rather than a thermal effect as used in the other treatment options is seen as the reason behind the large number of procedures being performed without general anaesthesia, although acceptability of anaesthesia was not a randomized outcome measure.

Other techniques (Photosensitization/ELITT™)

When added to many tissues, 5-aminolevulinic acid (ALA) results in the accumulation of sufficient quantities of the endogenous photosensitiser protoporphyrin IX. When exposed to activating light, this results in destruction of the tissue. Local internal application of ALA has also been used for selective endometrial ablation in animal model systems[53] and in human clinical studies.[54] This is not commercially available and evaluation has not progressed past the initial case reports.

The ELITT™ device utilises an intrauterine diode laser that scatters a laser beam around the endometrial cavity. It is a non-hysteroscopic method and purports the benefit of treating irregular cavities and difficult to access areas (such as the cornua) equally well.[55,56] A randomized controlled trial comparison of TCRE to ELITT™ has been reported[57] in which endometrial preparation in both arms was with GnRH agonists. At a 12-month follow-up 56% in the ELITT™ group and 23% in the TCRE group were amenorrhoeic. At 36 months, the figures were 61% for ELITT™ and 24% for TCRE. The data is encouraging, but at present the device is not commercially available.

Hysterectomy

Total hysterectomy is the only surgical treatment for menstrual problems that guarantees amenorrhoea. It is the most common surgical procedure in women in the UK, with 60 000 performed per annum. Hysterectomy rates are gradually falling, possibly because of improved techniques such as endometrial ablation and new effective medical treatments, in particular Mirena®. Satisfaction with hysterectomy is higher than that with ablation.[8] While effective, the procedure is not without risk and the complications of hysterectomy are often underestimated. Minor pyrexial morbidity was found in 47% of women after abdominal hysterectomy in the Pinion study,[58] with 11% having a vaginal vault haematoma and 5% requiring a blood transfusion. There were also three major complications in the same series.

The VALUE study in England, Wales and Northern Ireland is the most recent assessment of complications.[59] Unfortunately, unlike its sister publication the MISTLETOE study, the numbers included were a minority of the total number of procedures and there is a strong suspicion of a general under-reporting of cases and their complications.

The VALUE study assessed serious operative and postoperative complications (to 6 weeks) of hysterectomy in a prospective cohort of women undergoing hysterectomies for benign indications. A total of 37 512 women from 276 NHS and 145 private hospitals were studied. This group was originally recruited to compare the outcomes of endometrial destruction with those of hysterectomy. Severe operative complications occurred in 3%. The risk decreased with age and increased with greater parity and history of serious illness. Women with symptomatic fibroids experienced more complications than women with dysfunctional uterine bleeding, with an adjusted odds ratio of 1.3

(95% CI 1.1–1.6). Laparoscopic procedures doubled the risk of operative complications of abdominal hysterectomy giving an adjusted odds ratio of 1.9 (95% CI 1.5–2.5). Postoperative complications occurred in around 1% of women, showing a slight decrease with increasing age, and the strongest risk factor was a history of operative complications. Hysterectomies by the vaginal and laparoscopic route had significantly higher adjusted risks than abdominal operations (0.9%): RR = 1.4 (95% CI 1.0–1.9) and RR = 1.6 (95% CI 1.0–2.7). No intraoperative deaths were recorded. Within six weeks after surgery 14 women died giving a crude mortality rate of 3.8/1000 (range 2.5–6.4).

In the USA a large retrospective study of 1851 pre-menopausal women undergoing hysterectomy was undertaken.[60] The hysterectomies were performed by the abdominal route in 1283 women and vaginally in 568 women. The rate of fever after abdominal hysterectomy was 30% and 15% needed a blood transfusion. Vaginal hysterectomy had a lower rate of febrile morbidity of 15%. Bowel injury occurred in 3/1000 women following abdominal hysterectomy and 6/1000 after vaginal hysterectomy. The urinary tract was damaged in 3/1000 after abdominal hysterectomy but 14/1000 with the vaginal route. The mortality was 1/1000. A similar rate of bowel damage has been found in another large American study where the rate of bowel damage in abdominal gynaecological surgery has been reported as 8.4/1000 and 7.3/1000 for vaginal surgery.[14] Although the Dicker study advocated vaginal hysterectomy because of a 70% higher rate of complications after abdominal hysterectomy, the difference was mainly caused by relatively minor febrile problems and it was also not a randomized trial and thus the results are open to question. There was, however, more damage to the bowel or urinary tract during vaginal hysterectomy.[13]

LAPAROSCOPIC HYSTERECTOMY

Minimal access surgical techniques have been developed that allow for laparoscopic hysterectomy. The technique allows for varying levels of laparoscopic surgery from the division of upper pedicles (laparoscopic-assisted vaginal hysterectomy or LAVH), dissection and securing the uterine artery pedicle (laparoscopic hysterectomy), to a complete laparoscopic procedure (total laparoscopic hysterectomy) and allows for the addition of adnexal surgery and treatment of co-morbidities such as endometriosis. The technique has many exponents who extol the virtue of rapid recovery and minimal abdominal scarring. Randomized trial data from the eVALuate Trial exists to expand on the previous observational series.

Headed by Professor Ray Garry, the eVALuate trial group published the results of the largest trial of laparoscopic hysterectomy in 2004.[3] Two parallel multicentre trials were reported: the first trial comparing LAVH with abdominal hysterectomy in the abdominal trial, the second comparing LAVH with vaginal hysterectomy in the vaginal trial. The trial was multicentre looking at major complication as the primary outcome. Major complication was defined as: major haemorrhage (requiring transfusion); haematoma (requiring transfusion/surgical drainage); bowel, bladder, ureteric injury; pulmonary embolism; major anaesthetic complications; unintended laparotomy and wound dehiscence. A total of 1380 women were recruited with 1346 receiving surgery and 937 completing follow-up at 1 year.

Women were eligible if they required hysterectomy, had uteri 12 weeks in size or smaller and without significant prolapse (greater than first degree). The randomizing surgeon decided which arm – abdominal or vaginal – the patients entered into on clinical grounds. The laparoscopic procedures were a clinically heterogeneous group with LAVH, laparoscopic hysterectomy, laparoscopic supra-cervical hysterectomy and total laparoscopic hysterectomy included.

The conclusions of the trial were that laparoscopic surgery was associated with a significantly higher rate of major complications than abdominal surgery (unintended laparotomy and ureteric injury), took longer to perform (mean 84 minutes versus 50 minutes for abdominal and 79 minutes versus 39 minutes when compared with vaginal hysterectomy). Laparoscopic surgery was associated with faster recovery, less pain and better short-term quality of life.

A number of features of this trial deserve closer inspection and certain of these issues have been addressed in the *BJOG* editorial by Chien et al.[61] First, issues of generalisability arise. The allocation of patients into the abdominal or vaginal arm was made on clinical grounds. This allows the creation of allocation bias with the more potentially difficult cases being entered into the abdominal arm, thus skewing the complication rates in those randomised to laparoscopic hysterectomy.

Second is the definition of the primary outcome measure of major complication. The outcome measures were composite and could not be equally applied to each arm of the abdominal trial arm. An unintended laparotomy is not possible in the abdominal hysterectomy arm. The progress to open surgery for the laparoscopic arm may be seen as judicious surgery rather than a complication and if the complication rate was adjusted this would cast a much more favourable light over the laparoscopic arm's complication rate. If the complication rates are adjusted to exclude unintended laparotomy then the corrected incidences were not significantly different between the laparoscopic and abdominal arms (7.8% versus 6.2%, respectively).

Third, the individual surgeons in the trial were only required to have experience of 25 laparoscopic hysterectomies prior to inclusion. This does not represent the end of a learning curve[62] for laparoscopic surgery and this difference in experience may bias the results. This raises a training issue.

Fourth is the heterogeneous nature of the four laparoscopic procedures grouped together under the umbrella of 'laparoscopic hysterectomy'. The range of procedures varied from procedures that were the most technically challenging (a complete laparoscopic hysterectomy with all pedicles taken and the vagina opened laparoscopically) to the least invasive procedure (laparoscopic subtotal hysterectomy).

Overall, the validity of using a randomized controlled trial to address complication issues is questionable, as a study of this kind will always be underpowered to accurately comment on rates of complications. The trial does allow accurate estimation of effectiveness as measured by differences in quality-of-life scores. However the VALUE audit and the eVALuate trial also noted increased complications in those having laparoscopic hysterectomy when compared with those performed by other routes. Only 4% of hysterectomies are done by the laparoscopic route and these now tend to be done in centres where individuals have an interest and expertise in performing surgery by this route.

SUB-TOTAL HYSTERECTOMY

The first recorded hysterectomy was a subtotal procedure performed by Charles Clay in 1843.[63] This procedure remained the chosen method of abdominal hysterectomy for benign indications until the 1950s when the total abdominal hysterectomy predominated. In the 1980s a resurgence in the interest in sub-total hysterectomies occurred fuelled by the work on urinary and sexual function by Kilkku[64–66] and the emerging evidence of the long-term efficacy of the cervical screening programme. The procedure benefits from the reduced operative time and morbidity associated with preservation of the cervix uteri. A laparoscopic procedure is also possible.[67] The drawbacks of the procedure are the small numbers who will suffer from light bleeding/spotting from residual endometrial tissue high in the endocervical canal and the fear of cervical cancer in a cervical stump. Hysterectomy rates vary regionally and nationally, as do methods and the ratio of total abdominal hysterectomy to subtotal hysterectomy.[68,69] A significant decrease in total abdominal hysterectomy and an significant increase in the proportion of sub-total procedure is seen in the US data by Sills et al.[70] However, 99% still remain total abdominal procedures. Looking at national figures the Scandinavian countries have the highest ratio of sub-total to total procedures (the ratio in Sweden is 0.56) and the smallest reported ratio is in the UK (0.04).[69] A postal questionnaire of British gynaecologists reported in 1998 by Thakar et al. revealed subtotal hysterectomy to be an unpopular procedure in the UK, with 78% of female gynaecologists preferring a total hysterectomy for themselves.[71]

Comparisons between the total and subtotal procedure have been made with respect to a variety of outcomes. Urinary symptoms, bowel symptoms, pelvic organ prolapse and effects on sex life are assessed.

Overall it would appear that as a procedure sub-total hysterectomy has a lower blood loss than total, takes a shorter time to perform and has fewer perioperative (reduced rates of ureteric/bladder injury) and postoperative complications (especially pyrexia). On the downside it has a worse effect on bladder function than a total procedure and is associated with a not insignificant incidence of stump-related problems with 5%–20% of women having cyclical bleeding. There is no significant difference on the sexual function of patients post-total or sub-total hysterectomy. Intuitively one would think that pelvic organ prolapse would be less common after a subtotal procedure as the cervix retains the uterosacral and cardinal ligament complexes. The evidence points to no significant difference, but with a trend favouring total abdominal hysterectomy.[69]

OOPHORECTOMY AT HYSTERECTOMY

In general, healthy ovaries should be retained at hysterectomy and not routinely removed.[5] In women considering oophorectomy, the impact on the woman's health should be discussed (duration of hormone replacement therapy, effect on ischaemic heart disease risk, effect on ovarian/breast cancer risk, effect on libido). Oophorectomy should only be performed with the informed consent of the woman. It would be prudent in preoperative counselling to discuss and record the woman's wishes should unexpected ovarian pathology be encountered at hysterectomy. Women with a significant family history of ovarian or breast cancer should be seen by a geneticist to assess their risk and counsel them prior to considering prophylactic bilateral salpingo-oophorectomy. In women under 45 considering hysterectomy for heavy menstrual bleeding with other symptoms that may be related to ovarian dysfunction (for example, premenstrual syndrome), a trial of pharmaceutical ovarian suppression for at least 3 months should be used as a guide to the need for oophorectomy.[5]

Conclusion

A number of surgical procedures exist for the treatment of menstrual problems. Endometrial ablation is less invasive than hysterectomy, but requires further treatment in as many as 15%–25% of women; is not suitable for women with a cavity greater than 12 cm in size; is not contraceptive; and is associated with fewer complications and a quicker recovery than hysterectomy. Hysterectomy is very successful and associated with a high satisfaction rate; leads to a low but significant incidence of major complications, and minor complications are common; and can be performed by a number of routes depending on the surgeon's skills and the clinical scenario. When hysterectomy is performed for menstrual indications, healthy ovaries should be preserved.

References

1. Overton C, Hargreaves J, Maresh M. A national survey of the complications of endometrial destruction for menstrual disorders: the MISTLETOE study. Minimally Invasive Surgical Techniques – Laser, EndoThermal or Endorescetion. *Br J Obstet Gynaecol* 1997;104:1351–9.
2. A Scottish audit of hysteroscopic surgery for menorrhagia: complications and follow up. Scottish Hysteroscopy Audit Group. *Br J Obstet Gynaecol* 1995;102:249–54.
3. Garry R, Fountain J, Mason S, et al. The eVALuate study: two parallel randomised trials, one comparing laparoscopic with abdominal hysterectomy, the other comparing laparoscopic with vaginal hysterectomy. *BMJ* 2004;328:129.
4. Maresh MJ, Metcalfe MA, McPherson K, et al. The VALUE national hysterectomy study: description of the patients and their surgery. *BJOG* 2002;109:302–12.
5. National Collaborating Centre for Women's and Children's Health. *Heavy Menstrual Bleeding*. London: NICE; 2007 [http://www.nice.org.uk/cat.asp?c=63362].
6. Marjoribanks J, Lethaby A, Farquhar C. Surgery versus medical therapy for heavy menstrual bleeding. *Cochrane Database Syst Rev* 2006;(2):CD003855.
7. Lethaby A, Shepperd S, Cooke I, Farquhar C. Endometrial resection and ablation versus hysterectomy for heavy menstrual bleeding. *Cochrane Database Syst Rev* 2000;(2):CD000329.
8. Middleton LJ, Champaneria R, Daniels JP, et al. Hysterectomy, endometrial destruction, and levonorgestrel releasing intrauterine system (Mirena) for heavy menstrual bleeding: systematic review and meta-analysis of data from individual patients. *BMJ* 2010;341:c3929.
9. Goldrath MH, Fuller TA, Segal S. Laser photovaporization of endometrium for the treatment of menorrhagia. *Am J Obstet Gynecol* 1981;140:14–19.

10. Magos AL, Baumann R, Turnbull AC. Transcervical resection of the endometrium in women with menorrhagia. *BMJ* 1989;298:1209–12.
11. Gannon MJ, Holt EM, Fairbank J, et al. A randomised trial comparing endometrial resection and abdominal hysterectomy for the treatment of menorrhagia. *BMJ* 1991;303:1362–4.
12. Pinion SB, Kitchener HC, Parkin DE, Abramovich DR, Russell I, Alexander DA. Patient selection for hysteroscopic endometrial resection. *Br J Obstet Gynaecol* 1991;98:839.
13. Parkin DE. Prognostic factors for success of endometrial ablation and resection. *Lancet* 1998;351:1147–8.
14. Donnez J, Vilos G, Gannon MJ, Stampe-Sorensen S, Klinte I, Miller RM. Goserelin acetate (Zoladex) plus endometrial ablation for dysfunctional uterine bleeding: a large randomized, double-blind study. *Fertil Steril* 1997;68:29–36.
15. Rosenberg MK. Hyponatremic encephalopathy after rollerball endometrial ablation. *Anesth Analg* 1995;80:1046–8.
16. Arieff AI, Ayus JC. Endometrial ablation complicated by fatal hyponatremic encephalopathy. *JAMA* 1993;270:1230–2.
17. Bhattacharya S, Parkin DE, Reid TM, Abramovich DR, Mollison J, Kitchener HC. A prospective randomised study of the effects of prophylactic antibiotics on the incidence of bacteraemia following hysteroscopic surgery. *Eur J Obstet Gynecol Reprod Biol* 1995;63:37–40.
18. Parkin DE. Fatal toxic shock syndrome following endometrial resection. *Br J Obstet Gynaecol* 1995;102:163–4.
19. Crosignani PG, Vercellini P, Apolone G, De Giorgi O, Cortesi I, Meschia M. Endometrial resection versus vaginal hysterectomy for menorrhagia: long-term clinical and quality-of-life outcomes. *Am J Obstet Gynecol* 1997;177:95–101.
20. Dywer N, Hutton J, Stirrat GM. Randomised controlled trial comparing endometrial resection with abdominal hysterectomy for the surgical treatment of menorrhagia. *Br J Obstet Gynaecol* 1993;100:237–43.
21. O'Connor H, Broadbent JA, Magos AL, McPherson K. Medical Research Council randomised trial of endometrial resection versus hysterectomy in the management of menorrhagia. *Lancet* 1997;349:891–901.
22. Cooper KG, Jack SA, Parkin DE, Grant AM. Five-year follow up of women randomised to medical management or transcervical resection of the endometrium for heavy menstrual loss: clinical and quality of life outcomes. *BJOG* 2001;108:1222–8.
23. Kivnick S, Kanter MH. Bowel injury from rollerball ablation of the endometrium. *Obstet Gynecol* 1992;79:833–5.
24. Townsend DE. Bowel injury from rollerball ablation of the endometrium. *Obstet Gynecol* 1992;80:727.
25. Bhattacharya S, Cameron IM, Parkin DE, et al. A pragmatic randomised comparison of transcervical resection of the endometrium with endometrial laser ablation for the treatment of menorrhagia. *Br J Obstet Gynaecol* 1997;104:601–7.

26. Bae IH, Pagedas AC, Perkins HE, Bae DS. Postablation-tubal sterilization syndrome. *J Am Assoc Gynecol Laparosc* 1996;3:435–8.
27. Townsend DE, McCausland V, McCausland A, Fields G, Kauffman K. Post-ablation-tubal sterilization syndrome. *Obstet Gynecol* 1993; 82:422–4.
28. Webb JC, Bush MR, Wood MD, Park GS. Hematosalpinx with pelvic pain after endometrial ablation confirms the postablation-tubal sterilization syndrome. *J Am Assoc Gynecol Laparosc* 1996;3:419–21.
29. Cohen MM. Long-term risk of hysterectomy after tubal sterilization. *Am J Epidemiol* 1987;125:410–19.
30. Templeton AA, Cole S. Hysterectomy following sterilization. *Br J Obstet Gynaecol* 1982;89:845–8.
31. Cook JR, Seman EI. Pregnancy following endometrial ablation: case history and literature review. *Obstet Gynecol Surv* 2003;58:551–6.
32. Jack SA, Cooper KG, Graham W, Seymour J, Perez J. Office microwave endometrial ablation in the post menstrual phase – A RCT results to one year. *J Am Assoc Gynecol Laparosc* 2003;10:S4.
33. Marsh F, Thewlis J, Duffy S. Randomized controlled trial comparing Thermachoice III* in the outpatient versus daycase setting. *Fertil Steril* 2007;87:642–50.
34. Loffer FD. Three-year comparison of thermal balloon and rollerball ablation in treatment of menorrhagia. *J Am Assoc Gynecol Laparosc* 2001;8:48–54.
35. Loffer FD, Grainger D. Five-year follow-up of patients participating in a randomized trial of uterine balloon therapy versus rollerball ablation for treatment of menorrhagia. *J Am Assoc Gynecol Laparosc* 2002;9:429–35.
36. Meyer WR, Walsh BW, Grainger DA, Peacock LM, Loffer FD, Steege JF. Thermal balloon and rollerball ablation to treat menorrhagia: a multicenter comparison. *Obstet Gynecol* 1998;92:98–103.
37. Bain C, Cooper KG, Parkin DE. Microwave endometrial ablation versus endometrial resection: a randomized controlled trial. *Obstet Gynecol* 2002;99:983–7.
38. Cooper KG, Bain C, Parkin DE. Comparison of microwave endometrial ablation and transcervical resection of the endometrium for treatment of heavy menstrual loss: a randomised trial. *Lancet* 1999;354:1859–63.
39. Corson SL, Brill AI, Brooks PG, et al. One-year results of the vesta system for endometrial ablation. *J Am Assoc Gynecol Laparosc* 2000;7: 489–97.
40. Cooper J, Gimpelson R, Laberge P, et al. A randomized, multicenter trial of safety and efficacy of the NovaSure system in the treatment of menorrhagia. *J Am Assoc Gynecol Laparosc* 2002;9:418–28.
41. Duleba AJ, Heppard MC, Soderstrom RM, Townsend DE. A randomized study comparing endometrial cryoablation and rollerball electroablation for treatment of dysfunctional uterine bleeding. *J Am Assoc Gynecol Laparosc* 2003;10:17–26.

42. Corson SL. A multicenter evaluation of endometrial ablation by Hydro ThermAblator and rollerball for treatment of menorrhagia. *J Am Assoc Gynecol Laparosc* 2001;8:359–67.
43. Medical and Healthcare Products Regulatory Agency. *Medical Device Alert: Action Update. Devices Used for Endometrial Ablation. All Makes and Models.* London: MHRA; 2010 [http://www.mhra.gov.uk/Publications/Safetywarnings/MedicalDeviceAlerts/CON068319].
44. US Food and Drug Administration. Manufacturer and User Facility Device Experience Database (MAUDE) [http://www.accessdata.fda.gov/scripts/cdrh/cfdocs/cfMAUDE/search.CFM].
45. Pellicano M, Guida M, Acunzo G, Cirillo D, Bifulco G, Nappi C. Hysteroscopic transcervical endometrial resection versus thermal destruction for menorrhagia: a prospective randomized trial on satisfaction rate. *Am J Obstet Gynecol* 2002;187:545–50.
46. Cooper KG, Bain C, Lawrie L, Parkin DE. A randomised comparison of microwave endometrial ablation with transcervical resection of the endometrium; follow up at a minimum of five years. *BJOG* 2005;112(4):470–5.
47. Sambrook AM, Cooper KG, Campbell MK, Cook JA. Clinical outcomes from a randomised comparison of microwave endometrial ablation with thermal balloon endometrial ablation for the treatment of heavy menstrual bleeding. *BJOG* 2009;116:1038–45.
48. Gallinat A, Nugent W. NovaSure impedance-controlled system for endometrial ablation. *J Am Assoc Gynecol Laparosc* 2002;9:283–9.
49. Baker VL, Adamson GD. Threshold intrauterine perfusion pressures for intraperitoneal spill during hydrotubation and correlation with tubal adhesive disease. *Fertil Steril* 1995;64:1066–9.
50. Baker VL, Adamson GD. Minimum intrauterine pressure required for uterine distention. *J Am Assoc Gynecol Laparosc* 1998;5:51–3.
51. Dobak JD, Willems J. Extirpated uterine endometrial cryoablation with ultrasound visualization. *J Am Assoc Gynecol Laparosc* 2000;7:95–101.
52. Duleba AJ, Heppard MC, Soderstrom RM, Townsend DE. A randomized study comparing endometrial cryoablation and rollerball electroablation for treatment of dysfunctional uterine bleeding. *J Am Assoc Gynecol Laparosc* 2003;10:17–26.
53. Krzemien AA, Van Vugt DA, Pottier RH, Dickson EF, Reid RL. Evaluation of novel nonlaser light source for endometrial ablation using 5-aminolevulinic acid. *Lasers Surg Med* 1999;25:315–22.
54. Wyss P, Caduff R, Tadir Y, et al. Photodynamic endometrial ablation: morphological study. *Lasers Surg Med* 2003;32:305–9.
55. Donnez J, Polet R, Squifflet J, et al. Endometrial laser intrauterine thermotherapy (ELITT): a revolutionary new approach to the elimination of menorrhagia. *Curr Opin Obstet Gynecol* 1999;11:363–70.
56. Donnez J, Polet R, Rabinovitz R, Ak M, Squifflet J, Nisolle M. Endometrial laser intrauterine thermotherapy: the first series of 100 patients observed for 1 year. *Fertil Steril* 2000;74:791–6.

57. Perino A, Castelli A, Cucinella G, Biondo A, Pane A, Venezia R. A randomized comparison of endometrial laser intrauterine thermotherapy and hysteroscopic endometrial resection. *Fertil Steril* 2004;82:731–4.
58. Pinion SB, Parkin DE, Abramovich DR, et al. Randomised trial of hysterectomy, endometrial laser ablation, and transcervical endometrial resection for dysfunctional uterine bleeding. *BMJ* 1994;309:979–83.
59. McPherson K, Metcalfe MA, Herbert A, Maresh M, Casbard A, Hargreaves J, et al. Severe complications of hysterectomy: the VALUE study. *BJOG* 2004;111:688–94.
60. Dicker RC, Scally MJ, Greenspan JR, et al. Hysterectomy among women of reproductive age. Trends in the United States, 1970–1978. *JAMA* 1982;248:323–7.
61. Chien P, Khan K, Mol BW. How to interpret the findings of the eVALuate study. *BJOG* 2005;112:391–3.
62. Wattiez A, Soriano D, Cohen SB, et al. The learning curve of total laparoscopic hysterectomy: comparative analysis of 1647 cases. *J Am Assoc Gynecol Laparosc* 2002;9:339–45.
63. Leonardo RA. *History of Gynaecology*. New York: Foben Press; 1944.
64. Kilkku P. Supravaginal uterine amputation vs. hysterectomy. Effects on coital frequency and dyspareunia. *Acta Obstet Gynecol Scand* 1983;62:141–5.
65. Kilkku P, Grönroos M, Hirvonen T, Rauramo L. Supravaginal uterine amputation vs. hysterectomy. Effects on libido and orgasm. *Acta Obstet Gynecol Scand* 1983;62:147–52.
66. Kilkku P. Supravaginal uterine amputation versus hysterectomy with reference to subjective bladder symptoms and incontinence. *Acta Obstet Gynecol Scand* 1985;64:375–9.
67. Okaro EO, Jones KD, Sutton C. Long term outcome following laparoscopic supracervical hysterectomy. *BJOG* 2001;108:1017–20.
68. Baskett TF. Hysterectomy: evolution and trends. *Best Pract Res Clin Obstet Gynaecol* 2005;19:295–305.
69. Gimbel H. Total or subtotal hysterectomy – what is the evidence? In: Bonnar J, Dunlop W, editors. *Recent Advances in Obstetrics and Gynaecology*. London: Royal Society of Medicine Press; 2005. pp. 169–81.
70. Sills ES, Saini J, Steiner CA, McGee M III, Gretz HF III. Abdominal hysterectomy practice patterns in the United States. *Int J Gynaecol Obstet* 1998;63:277–83.
71. Thakar R, Manyonda I, Robinson G, Clarkson P, Stanton S. Total versus subtotal hysterectomy: a survey of current views and practice among British gynaecologists. *J Obstet Gynaecol* 1998;18:267–9.

6 Uterine fibroids and heavy menstrual bleeding

Uterine fibroids are the most common tumour of the female reproductive tract and occur in approximately 25% of women of reproductive age.[1] They are frequently asymptomatic but, when they do cause symptoms, these are likely to be menstrual problems, subfertility or symptoms associated with the size of the fibroids. It is still uncertain why fibroids cause menstrual problems; this is discussed below, together with a brief discussion of investigation.

Traditionally, treatment has been surgical: hysterectomy for those who have completed their childbearing and myomectomy for those who wish to retain their uterus. Surgery is associated with operative mortality and morbidity. Myomectomy may also be associated with a risk of hysterectomy, postoperative adhesion formation and recurrence. Until recently, many women have undergone hysterectomy even though they would have preferred a treatment that allowed them to maintain their fertility. It is for this reason that a number of options have been developed in recent years, as is discussed later in the chapter.

Diagnosis of fibroids

The only reason why fibroids can be treated conservatively without a tissue diagnosis is that malignancy is very unusual. It is almost impossible to determine an accurate incidence because the denominator is also unknown, since probably 50% of women are asymptomatic. In addition, leiomyosarcoma tends to occur in women in their 60s and 70s, whereas uterine fibroids occur in women of reproductive age.

Diagnosis is made by imaging, either ultrasound or magnetic resonance imaging (MRI) (Figure 6.1). MRI is particularly suitable for large fibroids and also allows the number of fibroids to be determined more easily than with ultrasound, although ultrasound, particularly with modern equipment, is very accurate for those with fibroids below about 10 cm in size. However, MRI also facilitates visualization of the ovaries, which can be difficult in women with large fibroids using ultrasound, and is superior in terms of identifying adenomyosis.

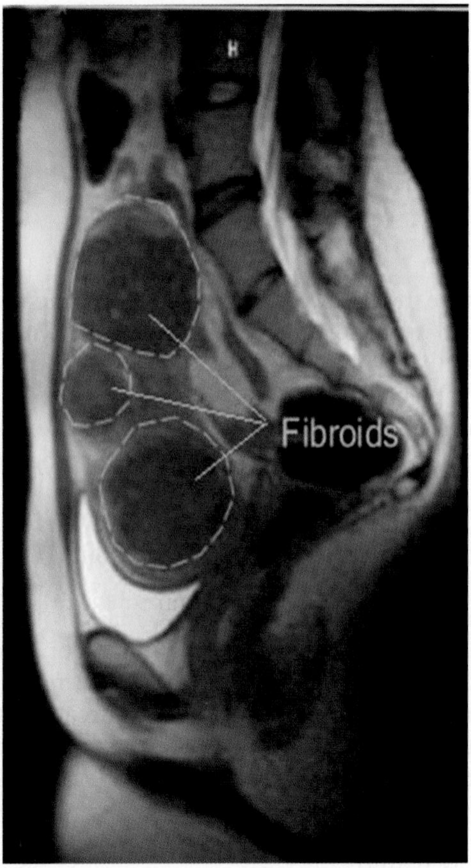

Figure 6.1 MRI showing uterine fibroids, courtesy of Professor Jon Moss, Gartnaval General Hospital, Glasgow

Fibroids and heavy menstrual bleeding

Women with uterine fibroids often complain of heavy menstrual bleeding (HMB). Epidemiological studies suggest that when women without fibroids complain of HMB, in fact only 40% will have a loss outside the normal range; however, with fibroids this is not the case and extremely heavy menstrual loss is much more common, frequently leading to anaemia.[2] This may be associated with other menstrual disorders such as intermenstrual bleeding or dysmenorrhoea.

Why fibroids cause bleeding is uncertain. It seems likely that it is most often associated with submucous fibroids although heavy loss in the presence of even subserous fibroids is documented.[3] Reasons why loss may be increased are:

- increased area or distortion of the uterine cavity
- abnormalities of blood supply of the uterus
- endometrial abnormalities
- ovulatory dysfunction (i.e. associated with both disorders of ovulation and increased oestrogen levels).

The most likely reason would seem to be distortion of the cavity and endometrial abnormalities. In regard to the latter, studies have suggested that various factors known to be associated with control of menstruation are found in abnormal quantities including:[4–6]

- prostaglandins
- growth factors (e.g. vascular endothelial growth factor)
- inflammatory mediators
- abnormalities of apoptosis.

However, it is difficult to be certain of their role and consequently more research is required.

Fibroids and fertility

For many years there was uncertainty as to whether fibroids did in fact cause infertility or were simply an association. Both fibroids and infertility are common in the older woman and in many instances fibroids are first diagnosed during pregnancy. However, data from assisted conception units indicate that the presence of submucous and possibly intramural fibroids leads to a decrease in implantation rates. Consequently, there is an argument for removing fibroids in women trying to conceive and who are experiencing difficulty. However, many of the studies are poor and do not take into account other complicating factors such as ovulatory disorders or male factors. A review of the literature suggests that more research in this area is desperately needed.[7]

Control of fibroid growth

Oestrogen is essential for fibroid growth. Gonadotrophin-releasing hormone (GnRH) agonists downregulate the pituitary with the subsequent decrease in estradiol levels leading to fibroid shrinkage.[8] Other studies suggest that progesterone and its receptor play a key role. The fibroid shrinkage that occurs with hypoestrogenism may be reversed by co-administration of synthetic progestins, although this is not a consistent finding across all studies. Progesterone receptor modulators have also been developed for use prior to surgery and potentially as a long-term medical treatment. These methods are discussed more fully below.

Treatment of fibroids

As mentioned above, treatment has often been surgical.[9]. Box 6.1 lists new treatments for uterine fibroids.

BOX 6.1 NEW TREATMENTS FOR UTERINE FIBROIDS

Medical treatment:

- Progesterone receptor modulators

Non-medical treatment:

- Uterine artery embolisation
- High-intensity focused ultrasound
- Ligation of the uterine arteries
- MRI-guided laser ablation

STANDARD TREATMENT OF FIBROIDS

Standard treatment consists of hysterectomy and myomectomy, the former being appropriate for those women who have completed their families. However, all surgery is associated with complications and the number of severe complications is increased in the presence of fibroids.[10,11] Both procedures may be carried out at laparotomy, although endoscopic procedures are now widely used. Hysterectomy is discussed in Chapter 4.

Myomectomy

Myomectomy is performed much less often than hysterectomy, with around one myomectomy to ten hysterectomies. Myomectomy can be carried out by laparotomy, laparoscopy or hysteroscopy depending on the size and number of the fibroids (see Figures 6.2 and 6.3).[12,13] There are no randomized controlled trials comparing myomectomy against no treatment, so efficacy is determined by 'before and after' studies. Myomectomy may improve fertility in some instances,

(a)

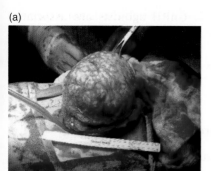

Figure 6.2a A fibroid being removed at abdominal myomectomy, courtesy of Dr David Parkin, Aberdeen Royal Infirmary

(b)

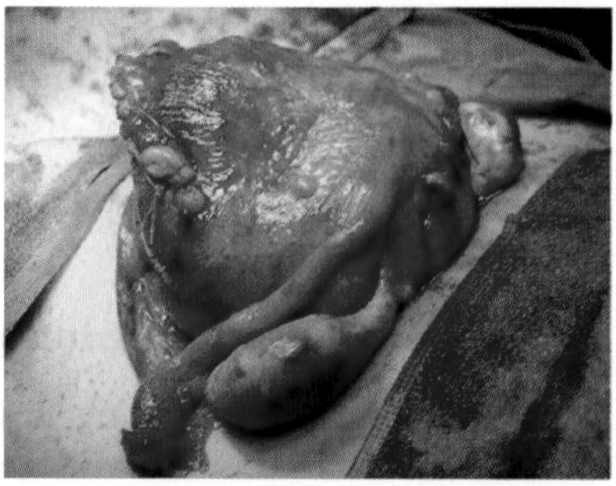

Figure 6.2b Suture line following removal of the fibroid in Figure 6.2a, courtesy of Dr David Parkin, Aberdeen Royal Infirmary

(a)

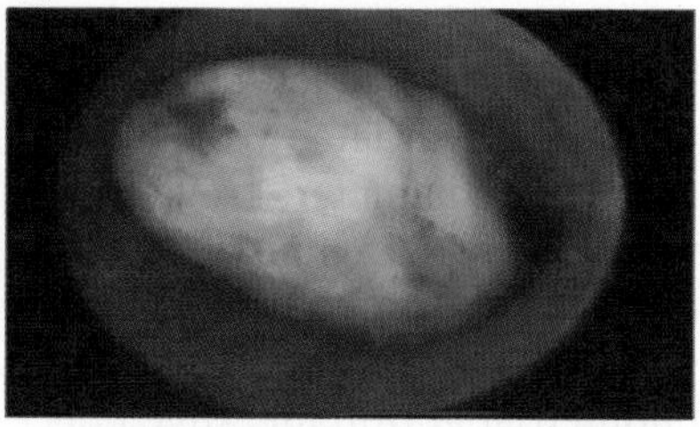

Figure 6.3a Hysteroscopic view of an intracavity fibroid

(b)

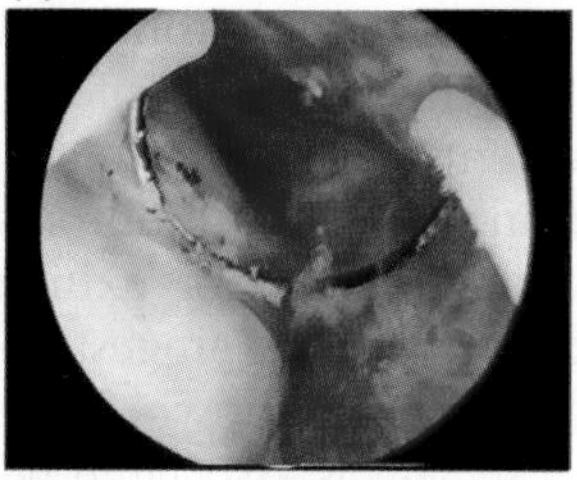

Figure 6.3b Uterine fibroid being removed using a resectoscope

although its relevance to the removal of subserosal fibroids is uncertain. The best data are from removal of submucosal fibroids, as is the case when myomectomy is performed to treat HMB. Myomectomy can be a challenging procedure if the fibroids are large or if the fibroids are in an unusual position and sometimes hysterectomy is required because of technical difficulty (usually bleeding). Since myomectomy is rather an unsatisfactory operation overall, new treatments are becoming available as some women do not wish to lose their uterus.

There is always a small risk of hysterectomy when myomectomy is carried out, particularly if the fibroids are large or are in an awkward position.

GnRH agonists may be used prior to surgery to shrink the fibroids.[8] GnRH agonists are usually given as a subcutaneous injection and downregulate the pituitary, with subsequent decrease in estradiol levels. This leads to a decrease in both the blood supply to the uterus and fibroid volume by about 50%. GnRH agonists are associated with postmenopausal-type adverse effects and are usually given for only 6 months, unless hormones are 'added back' to prevent the symptoms. However, their use is not generally considered to be cost-effective.

Levonorgestrel-secreting intrauterine system

The levonorgestrel-secreting intrauterine system is useful where fibroids are small and do not significantly distort the cavity. However, failure occurs in many cases with heavy menstrual loss since the expulsion rate is high and the efficacy uncertain.

Progesterone receptor modulators

The role of progesterone in the control of fibroid growth needs clarification. The presence of intrauterine progestogen does not have a consistent effect on fibroid size, although it is associated with relief of HMB in women with fibroids less than 4 cm in diameter. Progesterone receptor modulators exhibit partial and mixed agonist/antagonist effects on various progesterone target tissues in animals and humans and have been shown to be effective in decreasing menstrual blood loss.[22,23] This is associated with an endometrial antiproliferative effect, although ovarian function may not change. The histological findings have proved difficult to interpret, although they are not thought to represent an increased likelihood of malignancy.

Progesterone receptor modulators have been studied in women with uterine fibroids over a 3-month treatment period and have a dose-dependent effect leading to decreased menstrual blood loss in up to 83% of women. They also decrease uterine artery blood flow.

Progesterone receptor modulators have a modest effect on size which is not related to decreased menstrual blood loss. This means they are unlikely to be effective where fibroid size is the principal presenting complaint.

Progesterone receptor modulators:

- are effective
- improve menstrual problems
- improve quality of life
- have little impact on ovarian function
- are well tolerated.

The decrease in uterine artery blood flow also may contribute to the efficacy of other treatments for fibroid-related symptoms such as GnRH agonists, in addition to the decrease in fibroid size.[24,25] However, progesterone receptor modulators produce unusual effects on the endometrium that are difficult to interpret, which is limiting their long-term use. Recent publications[24,25] suggest that progesterone receptor modulators increase the haemoglobin when administered for 3 months preoperatively and, since they relieve menstrual problems during this period, may be used in this context in the same way as GnRH agonists.

When developed further, these drugs are likely to be very popular agents for use by women who wish to have conservative treatment for their uterine fibroids.

OTHER NEWER TREATMENTS FOR FIBROIDS

Uterine artery embolization

Uterine artery embolization (UAE) has been carried out for the treatment of uterine fibroids since 1995. The technique is illustrated in Figure 6.4. Prior to this, UAE was used for massive obstetric haemorrhage and also bleeding from organs such as the liver, which is

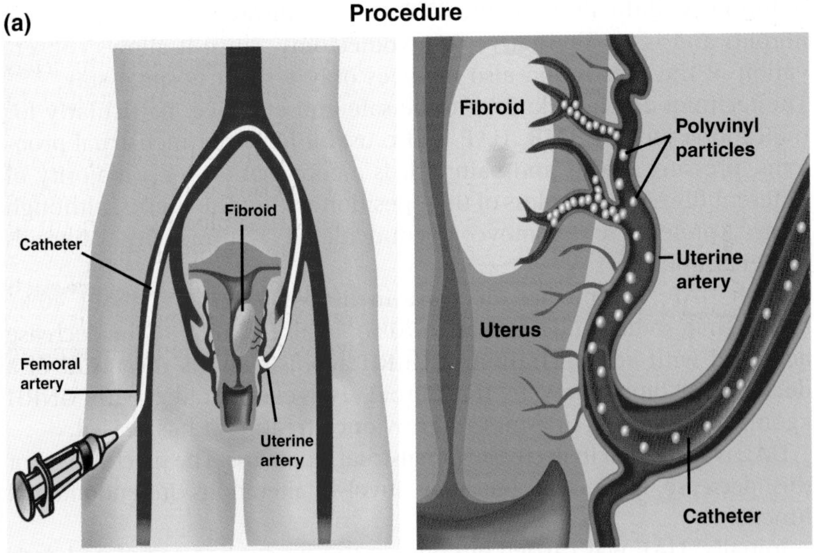

Figure 6.4a Uterine artery embolization: particles are injected through a cannula into the uterine artery via the femoral artery until flow stops

(b) Uterine artery embolization

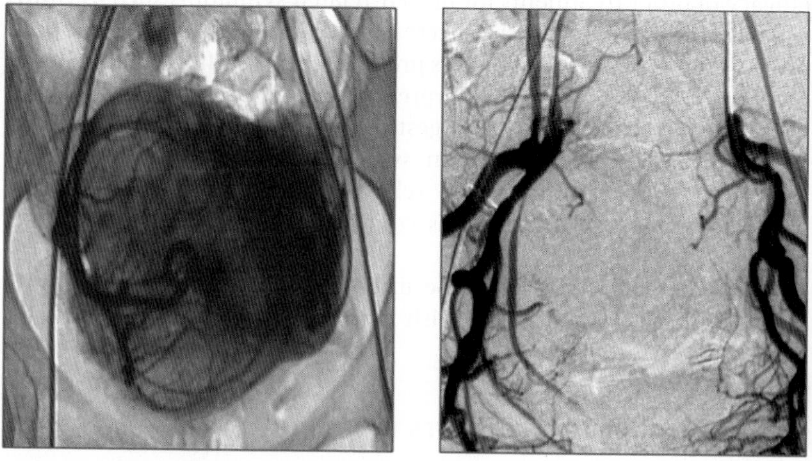

Image courtesy of Professor J Moss, Department of Radiology, Gartnaval General Hospital, Glasgow

Figure 6.4b Angiogram depicting the vessels to the fibroid before and after injection of particles

notoriously difficult to control. UAE is indicated for symptomatic fibroids and is an alternative to myomectomy, since it allows conservation of the uterus and also involves only a short hospital stay.[14–17] The technique is now known to be safe and effective, particularly for indications such as HMB. UAE is also useful for other menstrual problems, pressure effects and pain.[18] It is a good option for a majority of different fibroids regardless of their position within the uterus, although some prefer to remove pedunculated, intracavity fibroids hysteroscopically.

With UAE, the median decrease in fibroid volume is about 40%, although in some studies it is up to 70%.[18] This is similar to the decrease achieved with administration of GnRH agonists and is the result of a decrease in blood flow to the fibroid. However, unlike with GNRH agonists, the fibroid does not re-grow once treatment has ceased.

UAE is successful in decreasing menstrual blood loss. The mechanism for this decrease is unclear but may involve alterations in endometrial function.[5]

Initially, UAE was carried out only in those who had completed their families, but now it is felt that UAE can be used in women wishing to have a pregnancy in the future, although careful counselling is required. The counselling must cover the impact of UAE on ovarian function as well as the possibility of increased pregnancy complications.

The objective of UAE is to completely infarct all the fibroid tissue while preserving the uterus, ovaries and surrounding pelvic tissues. The procedure normally requires an overnight stay, since pain after UAE is a common problem but responds well to analgesia.

Data regarding complications are best obtained from the registries and large observational studies such as the HOPEFUL audit,[19,20] since the randomised controlled trials are not powered to show a difference in complication rates. Complications can be serious, although this is rarely the case, and can be divided as shown in Box 6.2.

BOX 6.2 COMPLICATIONS OF UAE

Immediate (occurring during the procedure):

- Haematoma, thrombosis or pseudoaneurism of femoral artery
- Reaction to the contrast media
- Procedural failure
- Excessive embolization
- Pain

Early (within the first 30 days):

- Vaginal discharge is common and usually settles down within a few days
- Postembolization syndrome (common but rarely severe), consisting of pain, nausea, an influenza-like illness, mild pyrexia and raised inflammatory markers
- Significant infection (rare)
- Continuing pain

Late (beyond 30 days)

Unlike with surgical treatment, some of the complications of UAE occur beyond 30 days or start earlier and continue beyond this time:

- Chronic vaginal discharge
- Fibroid expulsion
- Amenorrhoea (temporary amenorrhoea is common)
- Ovarian failure

UAE has been shown to be cost-effective, since the hospital stay is consistently shorter and recovery of normal milestones is rapid. UAE is a very useful proven uterine-sparing procedure, but success cannot be guaranteed. UAE is associated with a short recovery time and most women are very satisfied.

Data have emerged suggesting that there is an increase in pregnancy complications such as preterm labour and postpartum haemorrhage in women receiving UAE. However, unless the data are compared against women with untreated fibroids, they are difficult to interpret. The adverse effect of UAE on ovarian function appears to be related to age and is very uncommon in women under 40 years of age.[17,21]

High-intensity focused ultrasound

High-intensity focused ultrasound is a thermoablative technique that has been studied for over 60 years and has recently been recognized by NICE as being a safe and effective treatment for fibroids. In the past it has been used to treat tumours of the prostate, breast and liver and uses either ultrasound or MRI guidance.

MRI-guided focused ultrasound for uterine fibroids is a non-invasive thermoablative technique. As with diagnostic ultrasound, the waves pass through the anterior abdominal wall and significant heating occurs only where the waves converge at the focus. This allows treatment to be confined to the fibroid itself rather than involving surrounding myometrium.[26]

This technique provides continuous imaging not only of the fibroid but also of other surrounding vital structures such as bowel, bladder, and sacral nerves. It also allows the temperature of every treatment point to be monitored. Each therapeutic sonication is preceded by imaging of the treatment area and followed by temperature feedback in order that a surgeon can increase power if necessary to optimise effective calculation of the tissues. There is also the potential to prevent damage to other surrounding normal tissues.

Evaluation studies are being carried out looking at quality of life and the presenting symptoms of the fibroids. Data are promising, although the decrease in the size of the uterine fibroids seems to be modest compared with other treatment modalities.[27]

MRI-guided focused ultrasound appears to be a safe intervention with symptom improvement in many women.[28] It is limited by the fact that only a small number of fibroids can be treated in one session, and consequently those with multiple fibroids are either unsuitable or need to have multiple treatment sessions. At the moment the risk of recurrence is unclear and only long-term studies will be able to determine this. Although the volume reduction is small, symptom resolution can occur, possibly because of the alteration in the production of angiogenic growth factors from the myomas. This technique is also thought to be cost-effective.

As with UAE the initial clinical trials excluded women desiring pregnancy, although a study designed for women trying to conceive has been commenced and the results look promising.[29] Complications were common, but it is difficult to be sure whether the rate would be higher in a cohort of similar women not receiving the treatment.

Data are available at 12 and 24 months.[27] Outcome is directly related to the non-perfused volume of the fibroid, as might be expected, which impacts on the number of women requiring a repeat treatment. It is probable that, as experience of the technique grows, success will increase as more of the fibroid will be 'treated'. Long-term efficacy does not seem to be associated with a greater likelihood of adverse events. Sacral neuropathy has occurred, as have skin burns.

MRI-guided focused ultrasound is not readily available as the equipment is found in only a few centres around the world. However, this is a modality that is likely to develop and become important in the treatment of uterine fibroids. It has been compared with UAE and long-term results are awaited with interest.[29]

MRI-guided focused ultrasound can be performed as an outpatient procedure. It is associated with:

- local treatment of the fibroids with some shrinkage
- decreased menstrual blood loss
- improvement in quality of life
- no effect on ovarian function
- no increase in infection
- minimal discomfort
- little effect on pregnancy outcome
- unknown risk of recurrence.

Uterine artery occlusion

Gynaecologists who are experts in laparoscopic surgery might wish to carry out uterine artery occlusion to achieve relief of fibroid-related symptoms. The underlying mechanism is similar to that of UAE but uses external rather than internal occlusion. Studies of this procedure often include younger women and so outcomes are difficult to compare.

Conclusion

It is important to consider the position, size and number of the fibroids when making any comparison between treatment modalities. UAE and possibly the levonorgestrel-secreting intrauterine system are likely to be more suitable for women with multiple fibroids than MRI-guided focused ultrasound. None of these treatments is likely to be of value in women with large fibroids where size is the main symptom as the mean decrease in fibroid volume is less than 50% in most studies.

References

1. Buttram VC Jr, Reiter RC. Uterine leiomyomata: etiology, symptomatology, and management. *Fertil Steril* 1981;36:433–45.
2. Fraser IS, McGarron G, Markham R, Resta T, Watts A. Measured menstrual blood loss in women with pelvic disease or coagulation disorder. *Obstet Gynecol* 1986;68:630–3.
3. Sulaiman S, Khaund A, McMillan N, Moss J, Lumsden MA. Uterine fibroids – do size and location determine menstrual bloodloss? *Eur J Obstet Gynecol Reprod Biol* 2004;115:85–9.
4. Sinclair DC, Mastroyannis A, Taylor HS. Leiomyoma simultaneously impair endometrial BMP-2-mediated decidualization and anticoagulant expression through secretion of TGF-β3. *J Clin Endocrinol Metab* 2011;96:412–21.
5. Maybin JA, Critchley HO, Jabbour HN. Inflammatory pathways in endometrial disorders. *Mol Cell Endocrinol* 2011;335:42–51.
6. Kang JL, Wang DY, Wang XX, Yu J. Up-regulation of apoptosis by gonadotrophin-releasing hormone agonist in cultures of endometrial cells from women with symptomatic myomas. *Hum Reprod* 2010;25:2270–5.
7. Klatsky PC, Tran ND, Caughey AB, Fujimoto VY. Fibroids and reproductive outcomes: a systematic literature review from conception to delivery. *Am J Obstet Gynecol* 2008;198:357–66.
8. Lumsden MA, West CP, Thomas E, et al. Treatment with the gonadotrophin releasing hormone-agonist goserelin before hysterectomy for uterine fibroids. *BrJ Obstet Gynaecol* 1994;101:438–42.
9. Zimmermann A, Bernuit D, Gerlinger C, Schaefers M, Geppert K. Prevalence, symptoms and management of uterine fibroids: an international internet-based survey of 21,746 women. *BMC Womens Health* 2012;12:6.
10. Maresh M, Metcalfe MA, McPherson K, et al. The VALUE national hysterectomy study: description of the patients and their surgery. *BJOG* 2002;109:302–12.
11. McPherson K, Metcalfe MA, Herbert A, et al. Severe complications of hysterectomy: the VALUE study. *BJOG* 2004;111:688–94.
12. Lumsden MA. Modern management of fibroids. *Obstet Gynaecol Reprod Med* 2010;20:82–6.

13. Wen KC, Sung MD, Chao KC, Lee WL, Liu WM, Wang PH. A prospective short-term evaluation of uterine leiomyomas treated by myomectomy through conventional laparotomy or ultraminilaparotomy. *Fertil Steril* 2008;90:2361–6.
14. van der Kooij SM, Bipat S, Hehenkamp WJ, Ankurn WM, Reckers JA. Uterine artery embolization versus surgery in the treatment of symptomatic fibroids: a systematic review and metaanalysis. *Am J Obstet Gynecol* 2011;205:317.e1–18.
15. Edwards RD, Moss JG, Lumsden MA, et al.; Committee of the Randomized Trial of Embolization versus Surgical Treatment of Fibroids. Uterine-artery embolization versus surgery for symptomatic uterine fibroids. *N Engl J Med* 2007;356:360–70.
16. van der Kooij SM, Hehenkamp WJ, Volkers NA, Birnie E, Ankum WA, Reekers JA. Uterine artery embolization vs hysterectomy in the treatment of symptomatic uterine fibroids: 5-year outcome from the randomized EMMY trial. *Am J Obstet Gynecol* 2010;203:105.e1–13.
17. Moss JG, Cooper KG, Khaund A, et al. Randomised comparison of uterine artery embolisation (UAE) with surgical treatment in patients with symptomatic uterine fibroids (REST trial): 5-year results. *BJOG* 2011;118:936–44.
18. Khaund A, Moss JG, McMillan N, Lumsden MA. Evaluation of the effect of uterine artery embolisation on menstrual blood loss and uterine volume. *BJOG* 2004;111:700–5.
19. Hirst A, Dutton S, Wu O, et al. A multi-centre retrospective cohort study comparing the efficacy, safety and cost-effectiveness of hysterectomy and uterine artery embolisation for the treatment of symptomatic uterine fibroids. The HOPEFUL study. *Health Technol Assess* 2008;12:1–248, iii.
20. Dutton S, Hirst A, McPherson K, Nicholson T, Maresh M. A UK multicentre retrospective cohort study comparing hysterectomy and uterine artery embolisation for the treatment of symptomatic uterine fibroids (HOPEFUL study): main results on medium-term safety and efficacy. *BJOG* 2007;114:1340–51.
21. Rashid S, Khaund A, Murray LS, et al. The effects of uterine artery embolisation and surgical treatment on ovarian function in woman with uterine fibroids. *BJOG* 2010;117:985–9.
22. Bouchard P, Chabbert-Buffet N, Fauser BC. Selective progesterone receptor modulators in reproductive medicine: pharmacology, clinical efficacy and safety. *Fertil Steril* 2011;96:1175–89.
23. Wilkins J, Chwalisz K, Han C, et al. Effects of the selective progesterone receptor modulator asoprisnil on uterine artery blood flow, ovarian activity, and clinical symptoms in patients with uterine leiomyomata scheduled for hysterectomy. *J Clin Endocrinol & Metabol* 2008;93:4664–71.
24. Donnez J, Tatarchuk TF, Bouchard P, et al.; PEARL I Study Group. Ulipristal acetate versus placebo for fibroid treatment before surgery. *N Engl J Med* 2012;366:409–20.

25. Donnez J, Tomaszewski J, Vázquez F, et al.; PEARL II Study Group. Ulipristal acetate versus leuprolide acetate for uterine fibroids. *N Engl J Med* 2012;366:421–32.
26. Hudson SB, Stewart EA. Magnetic resonance-guided focused ultrasound surgery. *Clin Obstet Gynecol* 2008;51:159–66.
27. Gorny KR, Woodrum DA, Brown DL, et al. Magnetic resonance-guided focused ultrasound of uterine leiomyomas: review of a 12-month outcome of 130 clinical patients. *J Vasc Interv Radiol* 2011;22:857–64.
28. Bouwsma EV, Gorny KR, Hesley GK, Jensen JR, Peterson LG, Stewart EA. Magnetic resonance-guided focused ultrasound surgery for leiomyoma-associated infertility. *Fertil Steril* 2011;96:e9–e12.
29. Bouwsma EV, Hesley GK, Woodrum DA, et al. Comparing focused ultrasound and uterine artery embolization for uterine fibroids-rationale and design of the Fibroid Interventions: reducing symptoms today and tomorrow (FIRSTT) trial. *Fertil Steril* 2011;96:704–10.

7 Dysmenorrhoea

Dysmenorrhoea is common and many women consider it to be a normal part of menstruation. However, for some, pain is severe and life can be completely disrupted by their period. It is the most common cause of school absenteeism in teenage girls and may lead to the loss of a job through repeated days off work. For other women it is no more than a mild inconvenience. It is important to establish the impact on the woman's life during the initial assessment.

Women are sometimes surprisingly uncomplaining about the degree of disruption their periods are causing. Perhaps having grown up for years with a certain degree of pain, they consider it to be normal. However, if a patient brings the symptom to the doctor for help, their pain should never be dismissed.

Definition and epidemiology

Dysmenorrhoea is defined as painful cramps associated exclusively with menstrual bleeding. Estimates of its prevalence vary from 45%–95% of women and this is likely to reflect a wide range of pain severity.[1] It is thought that 2%–5% of women may suffer from severe dysmenorrhoea. Perhaps 20% may be affected by significantly disruptive pain.[2] Smoking is associated with dysmenorrhoea. Prevalence is inversely proportional to parity, but when parity is controlled for, age does not correlate with dysmenorrhoea.[3]

Traditionally, dysmenorrhoea has been classified as primary or secondary, depending whether associated pathology has been identified or not. Primary dysmenorrhoea describes pain which develops with or shortly before the onset of menstruation, and fades after the first day or two. It is said to begin shortly after menarche and is not associated with other symptoms or signs. It implies that teenagers who suffer with pain are less likely to have demonstrable pathology than an older woman experiencing a change in her usual level of pain. However this distinction may be difficult to defend, since many older women presenting for investigation describe their pain as having begun in their teens and gradually worsened to include additional symptoms and lengthening duration of symptoms. The distinction also relies on the women presenting to be investigated and on the certainty with which pathology has been excluded.

Potential causes of dysmenorrhoea

For a teenager, congenital uterine abnormalities may present with dysmenorrhoea. An imperforate hymen is likely to present with cyclical pain but no bleeding. However, if a non-communicating horn is present, the girl will have started to menstruate from the open horn, but a haematocolpos may be developing on the non-communicating side. An abdominal ultrasound would rule this out.

Endometriosis is the most common identifiable pathology associated with dysmenorrhoea. This is discussed in greater detail in Chapter 8. It certainly can present in adolescence, although often women are not diagnosed until their twenties or later. Adenomyosis is a related condition in which endometrioid tissue extends into the myometrium. It causes pain and possibly menstrual irregularity. For both these conditions, the diagnosis is essentially a clinical one based on the cyclicity of the pain. Diagnostic laparoscopy can be done in an attempt to identify endometriosis but the degree of pain bears little or no relation to the extent of disease seen at laparoscopy. Adenomyosis is not visible at laparoscopy. Laparoscopy also carries a significant surgical and anaesthetic risk, and may not be justifiable in an otherwise healthy woman. Magnetic resonance imaging (MRI) can be used to image adenomyosis, but again it is not a perfectly sensitive investigation.

If endometriosis or adenomyosis is present the important issue is control of symptoms. The disease is a chronic condition, which is likely to come and go during the woman's reproductive life, but cannot be eradicated except with hysterectomy and, possibly, removal of the ovaries. Some women will, very reasonably, be concerned that if endometriosis is present, their fertility may be adversely affected. If a woman is currently finding it difficult to conceive, particularly if dyspareunia is also present, it may be appropriate to perform a laparoscopy and dye test to explore the tubes and specifically to establish the degree of pelvic damage related to endometriosis, if any. It may also be possible to treat the endometriosis surgically at that point to reduce the woman's symptoms. The presence of endometriosis-related damage may affect her choices regarding the management of her fertility. With regard to the pain of endometriosis however, it is considered that although the disease may progress, potential damage to a woman's fertility cannot be prevented using medical or surgical treatment. Consequently there may be no advantage in making a laparoscopic diagnosis sooner rather than later for a woman who is not currently trying to conceive.

Pelvic infection may cause pain and bleeding, but would be an unlikely cause of chronic dysmenorrhoea alone. However, sexually transmitted infection (STI) is common, damaging and transmissible. Therefore there should be a low threshold for taking swabs in any young woman presenting with gynaecological symptoms. Upper genital tract infection, known as PID may cause damage leading to chronic pelvic pain (CPP) which may be principally associated with menstruation. Again, the important thing is to rule out an ongoing infection in the cervix which can be done by taking swabs.

For the older woman, fibroids may have developed, and particularly depending on their size and site, they may contribute to dysmenorrhoea. Fibroids are commonly asymptomatic.

In the absence of pathology, researchers have sought evidence of abnormal pain mediators in the uterus to account for increased pain. These factors may also be at work in the presence of identifiable pathology such as endometriosis. Prostaglandins have been identified in higher concentrations within the uterus and menstrual fluid in women suffering from dysmenorrhoea than in controls. It is thought that this may lead to a state of uterine hypertonicity, resulting either in myometrial waves of greater intensity or in higher resting tone. Uterine contractions may then lead to a degree of ischaemia, which may be the origin of the pain itself. Leucotrienes have also been demonstrated in increased concentrations in women with dysmenorrhoea and may have an inflammatory role.[4]

Assessing the patient

At the initial consultation an assessment should be made of the severity of pain and the level of disruption caused. The nature and pattern of the pain should be established. Dysmenorrhoea may begin a few hours before the onset of bleeding, but should tail away as the bleeding ends, or before. It is usually cramping in nature but may be constant. It may be felt in the suprapubic area and extend onto the tops of the thighs. It may also be referred to one or other iliac fossa or into the back. Pain affecting the rest of the menstrual cycle or radiating in a different pattern may suggest additional pathology. It may be helpful to know whether the woman has always suffered from dysmenorrhoea or whether it is of more recent onset.

The pattern and heaviness of bleeding should be established. The cycles may be regular or irregular or there may be chaotic bleeding with no underlying pattern to it. Particularly in an older woman, a recent change in the pattern of bleeding, such as intermenstrual bleeding or postcoital bleeding may warrant further investigation to exclude serious pathology such as endometrial or cervical carcinoma. Irregular menstruation may suggest anovulatory cycles, which may be heavier and consequently more painful. Heavy menstrual bleeding is common and is discussed in Chapter 1, but may need to be taken into account in planning treatment.

Other symptoms should be established as they might suggest other pathology or the need for further investigation. For example, although diarrhoea at the onset of menstruation is common, altered bowel habit throughout the cycle might suggest an element of irritable bowel syndrome which could be addressed specifically. Rectal pain or bleeding may suggest recto-vaginal endometriosis and specific enquiry should be made. Dyspareunia is also an important symptom and may be difficult for a woman to bring up unprompted. Vaginal discharge might suggest infection.

It is important to know about previous pregnancies and indeed to rule out a current pregnancy if appropriate. Enquiries should be made about future fertility plans. Contraception may be required in addition to treatment of the dysmenorrhoea. Alternatively, the woman may want to conceive and indeed the delay in conceiving may have actually prompted her visit. Investigation and treatment should be planned accordingly.

Many women will have tried self-medication to manage their pain. If new treatment is to be initiated it is useful to know what has already been tried.

An examination should be performed, although for a young woman, particularly if she is not sexually active, abdominal examination is usually sufficient. An abdominal mass should be ruled out and abdominal tenderness should be excluded.

If a vaginal examination is to be performed, the size, mobility and tenderness of the uterus should be established along with the presence of any pelvic masses, which might suggest endometriomas or fibroids. Nodularity may be found in the uterosacral ligaments or in the posterior fornix, again suggestive of endometriosis. If there is any possibility of STI, swabs should be taken. An opportunistic smear should be taken if the woman is not up to date or if there is clinical concern.

Investigation

Swabs should be taken to rule out infection if appropriate. An ultrasound may be helpful if the examination suggests pathology or if the patient has a particular concern (for example, fear of the presence of an ovarian cyst). If there are no other symptoms of concern and the examination is normal, no further investigation is required before initiating treatment. If on the other hand, the woman has concerns about her fertility, additional symptoms are present or medical treatment has failed, she may wish to consider a diagnostic laparoscopy specifically to look for endometriosis.

Management

If the woman wishes to avoid the use of hormones, perhaps because she wants to become pregnant, NSAIDs offer effective treatment. No particular NSAID can be recommended above another but an individual may get more benefit from one than another and therefore may wish to try more than one.[5] Starting to take the NSAID in the 24 hours before the onset of pain may increase its effectiveness. Paracetamol and codeine may be used in addition. Used regularly in combination with NSAIDs, these may be sufficient to control the pain, allowing normal function to be maintained even for women with severe dysmenorrhoea.

There is some evidence that physical remedies such as heat and transcutaneous electrical nerve stimulation (TENS) may be helpful.[6,7] Acupuncture, behavioural interventions, exercise and Chinese or herbal remedies have all been tried and to some extent evaluated in individual Cochrane reviews. Although evidence of benefit is lacking, if the woman finds that these interventions help her to cope, then they are of value. Women should be aware that some remedies may have adverse effects and may interact with other drugs.

If contraception is required, the levonorgestrel–secreting IUS offers excellent pregnancy prevention in addition to reduction in menstrual flow. This often leads to a reduction in pain but it is not licensed for this indication. Women must be warned about the irregular bleeding which most women experience at first, but with prolonged use the majority of women will experience amenorrhoea. Some women also experience progestogen-related side effects initially. Other forms of long-acting progestogen such as the Nexplanon® (Schering-Plough, Welwyn Garden City, Herts) or Depo-Provera® may be used, but these may be associated with higher rates of irregular or unscheduled bleeding. Because of its size the LNG–IUS may not be suitable for many teenagers and some older nulliparous women.

The combined oestrogen-containing pill also offers good contraception and substantial reduction in dysmenorrhoea.[8] The pill may be particularly helpful if the menstrual cycle is chaotic due to anovulatory cycles. It can be expected to both lighten and regulate the bleed as well as reduce pain. A progestogen – only contraceptive may be a useful alternative in women who cannot tolerate estrogen.

If symptoms are particularly troublesome and the woman wishes to stop the bleeding all together, she may choose high-dose progestogens or a GnRH analogue. Although these drugs have significant side effects and are not suitable for long-term use, it may allow the woman to get a break from the repeated disruption and make longer-term decisions. The use of these drugs is described in more detail in Chapter 3.

Ultimately, if the woman does not want to have any further children and feels that the symptoms are sufficiently severe to justify it, a hysterectomy may be the right choice for her. Some women may benefit from removal of the ovaries since retaining them may result in cyclical pain after the uterus alone is removed. The explanation for this is not clear but may represent remaining endometriotic tissue (visible or microscopic) which is sustained by the endogenous estrogen. Alternatively the ovaries may become encased in adhesions following hysterectomy which leads to cyclical pain. This is known as the retained ovary syndrome.

Surgical interruption of the nerve pathways supplying the uterus has been considered. Laparoscopic uterosacral nerve ablation (LUNA) is considered to be ineffective. Presacral neurectomy has been shown to be effective in the management of central severe dysmenorrhoea, but is potentially hazardous, with significant adverse effects on bladder and bowel function. It should only be undertaken by specialists in the field with full consent.[9]

Conclusions

Dysmenorrhoea is common and readily treatable. It may suggest underlying pathology, but if no additional sinister symptoms are present and other symptoms are well controlled with medical treatment, no further investigation is necessary provided the patient's concerns have been addressed.

Information for patients

Clinical knowledge summary: www.cks.nhs.uk/dysmenorrhoea.

References

1. Proctor M, Farquhar C. Diagnosis and management of dysmenorrhoea. *BMJ* 2006;332:1134–8.
2. Weissman AM, Hartz AJ, Hansen MD, Johnson SR. The natural history of primary dysmenorrhoea: a longitudinal study. *BJOG* 2004;111:345–52.

3. Sundell G, Milsom I, Andersch B. Factors influencing the prevalence and severity of dysmenorrhoea in young women. *Br J Obstet Gyn* 1990;97:588–94.
4. Harel Z. Dysmenorrhoea in adolescents and young adults: from pathophysiology to pharmacological treatments and management strategies. *Expert Opin Pharmacother* 2008;9:2661–72.
5. Marjoribanks J, Proctor ML, Farquhar C. Nonsteroidal anti-inflammatory drugs for primary dysmenorrhoea. *Cochrane Database Syst Rev* 2010;(1): CD001751.
6. Akin MD, Weingand KW, Hengehold DA, Goodale MB, Hinkle RT, Smith RP. Continuous low-level topical heat in the treatment of dysmenorrhoea. *Obstet Gynecol* 2001;97:343–9.
7. Proctor ML, Smith CA, Farquhar CM, Stones RW. Transcutaneous electrical nerve stimulation and acupuncture for primary dysmenorrhoea. *Cochrane Database Syst Rev* 2002;(1):CD002123.
8. Wong CL, Farquhar CM, Roberts H, Proctor ML. Oral contraceptive pill for primary dysmenorrhoea. *Cochrane Database Syst Rev* 2009;(4):CD002120.
9. Proctor M, Latthe P, Farquhar CM, Khan KS, Johnson NP. Surgical interruption of pelvic nerve pathways for primary and secondary dysmenorrhoea. *Cochrane Database Syst Rev* 2005;(4):CD001896.

Further reading

Dawood MY. Primary dysmenorrhoea: advances in pathogenesis and management. *Obstet Gynecol* 2006;108:428–41.

8 Endometriosis

Endometriosis is a common disease affecting approximately 10% of the female population.[1] It describes the presence of endometrioid tissue outside the cavity of the uterus. While endometriosis can be asymptomatic, it may lead to pain or subfertility. Many women experience severely disabling symptoms for many years before finding relief. Numerous questions still surround endometriosis – its pathophysiology, its natural history, the best method of diagnosis and the correct management. However, an explanation of the symptoms and effective treatment can be achieved for most sufferers, allowing them to return to normal function. It is important that this easily delivered support becomes more readily accessible to women in the future in order to reduce distress and disability.

Nature of endometriosis

Endometriosis is a hormone-dependent, inflammatory condition characterised by the presence of endometrioid tissue outside the uterus. Although it can occur in a number of forms, histologically it contains glandular elements and may produce a local inflammatory or fibrotic response in surrounding tissues. Some authorities consider the different forms to be different disease entities.

In its simplest form, endometriosis may exist as peritoneal disease, seen as deposits on an otherwise healthy peritoneum. These may have a variety of appearances: blue-black lesions, haemorrhagic areas, neovascularisation, lacunae formation or vesicles. Endometriosis may result in the formation of ovarian cysts, known as endometriomas. These are either within the ovary or trapped between the ovary and the pelvic side wall. The cysts are lined with endometrioid tissue which bleeds, leading to a fluid-filled cavity, which may enlarge over time. Endometriomas may be associated with extensive fibrosis. The fluid is altered blood and looks like molten chocolate, leading to the alternative name of 'chocolate cyst'.

Endometriosis may occur as nodules below the peritoneal surface, often associated with extensive fibrosis. The term deeply infiltrating endometriosis has been coined. Solid, fibrous nodules, at times 2–3 cm or more in diameter, can form below the peritoneal surface particularly in the pouch of Douglas. These can be difficult to visualize laparoscopically. The distortion associated with the fibrosis may affect the surrounding nerves and this distortion may itself lead to neuropathic pain.

Endometrioid tissue in the myometrium itself has been termed adenomyosis. It may share some characteristics of endometriosis or be a distinct disease. Only recently diagnosable through the development of MRI, understanding of this disease is limited, but it is thought to produce cyclical pain and infertility and perhaps abnormal menstrual bleeding as well.

Aetiology

Two major theories regarding the aetiology of endometriosis have been discussed for over 80 years. The first proposes that endometriosis arose as a result of retrograde menstruation (known to occur in most women normally) followed by seeding of viable endometrioid cells in dependent areas of the pelvis. Whereas for most women the immune system would clear away these stray cells, women with endometriosis are postulated to have either an immune defect which allows the proliferation of these ectopic cells or changes in the normal endometrium that promote the persistence of these ectopic deposits. Viable cells may disseminate through the body to distant sites by passing through the blood or lymphatic system. The alternative theory of coelomic metaplasia states that areas of embryological mesodermal cells undergo metaplasia leading to development of endometrioid cells in new sites not necessarily connected to the pelvis at all. Neither of these theories adequately explains the pattern of endometriosis observed in practice. For example, endometriosis has been observed in sites distant to the pelvis such as the brain and even rarely in cisgender men. This could not be explained by retrograde menstruation.

Recent research has examined the nature of the endometrioid tissue itself noting the production of chemicals such as interleukins, tumour necrosis factor and prostaglandins, which are potent pain mediators. Chemokines and cytokines provoke an inflammatory response associated with increased numbers of macrophages, granulocytes and natural killer cells. Altered hormone production has been observed, with high activity of aromatases within the endometrioid tissue, leading to greatly increased local oestrogen concentrations compared to eutopic endometrium. Data also point to increased nerve proliferation in endometrioid tissue. These observations may ultimately lead to a better understanding of the pathogenesis of endometriosis, and to the development of new therapeutic options. However, for the time being the aetiology of endometriosis has not been fully characterized.[2]

Symptoms of endometriosis

While endometriosis can be asymptomatic, two main groups of symptoms have been ascribed to the condition: pain and subfertility. However, the link between these symptoms and the extent of the disease is inconsistent and poorly understood.

The pain of endometriosis is said to vary with the menstrual cycle although it can be present to some extent every day. The triad of dysmenorrhoea (pain with menstruation), dyspareunia (pain on intercourse) and non-menstrual pelvic pain is considered characteristic. One difficulty in linking symptoms to diagnosis is that the diagnosis of endometriosis at laparoscopy, albeit considered the gold standard, may be imperfect.

Dyschezia (pain on opening the bowels) can be a feature of endometriosis and is sometimes overlooked by the woman or her doctor as not being relevant to her other symptoms. It can be extremely distressing – women describe a knife-like pain shooting up the rectum, making them unwilling or unable to open their bowels during menstruation. Rectal bleeding may also be present and can be profuse. It is important to enquire specifically about the bowels, as these symptoms may point towards rectovaginal endometriosis or bowel involvement. Alternatively they may of course be due to another cause such as an anal fissure, perhaps secondary to constipation, which should be identified and treated.

Women commonly describe other symptoms associated with their disease, which when the endometriosis is treated, tend to resolve. A myriad of symptoms have been described including malaise, headaches, nausea, bloating, diarrhoea, urinary frequency and many others. Given the paucity of our understanding of the disease, it behoves the clinician to take these seriously rather than dismiss the woman's own formulation out of hand. As our understanding of endometriosis improves, some of these symptoms can be understood as part of the expected symptom complex of endometriosis.

Pelvic pain is of course not always due to endometriosis and it is important to take a thorough history at the outset aiming to make a positive diagnosis of endometriosis or identify other factors such as musculoskeletal pain or irritable bowel syndrome. Care at the start of a woman's presentation may help to avoid fruitless investigations and years of frustrating misdiagnoses for the patient and the health service. The social and economic burden of untreated pain is vast. See Chapter 9 for a fuller discussion.

The link between subfertility and endometriosis is even harder to clarify. A diagnosis of endometriosis is more prevalent in the subfertile population than in the general population and women with diagnosed endometriosis are more likely to suffer difficulties in conceiving than other women.[3] However, many women with endometriosis, even with marked structural damage, go on to conceive spontaneously.

Various effects of endometriosis may explain subfertility. Where extensive adhesion formation has occurred, the tubes and surrounding structures may be severely distorted leading to tubal blockage and hydrosalpinges. Endometriomas may damage the ovary, either by a pressure effect or by the presence of toxic substances, leading to loss of ovarian reserve. This may be irreversible. Peritoneal disease even with no distortion of the pelvis also seems to reduce fertility, perhaps due to the presence of substances unfavourable to conception or toxic to eggs or sperm. Finally endometriosis may cause dyspareunia, which is likely to reduce the chances of conception, particularly if present around the time of ovulation.

Diagnosis

The gold standard for diagnosis has traditionally been diagnostic laparoscopy. This involves a general anaesthetic plus surgical risks that include a 1 in 500 risk of bowel damage.[4] The diagnosis is usually a visual one, but some authorities recommend routine peritoneal biopsy to confirm the diagnosis.[5] Laparoscopists vary in the extent to which they confidently label specific appearances as endometriosis. Evidence of fibrosis and adhesion formation may be easier to identify as clearly abnormal, but the origin of the damage may be unclear as previous infection or surgery may lead to adhesion formation in the absence of endometriosis. The presence of endometriomas is of course pathognomonic of endometriosis. Endometriomas can be readily treated at laparoscopy. It may be wise to at least biopsy these lesions to confirm that no malignant change is present. Nodules of endometriosis, particularly in the rectovaginal space can be difficult to detect laparoscopically, as only a pinpoint may be visible at the peritoneal surface. Careful vaginal and possibly also rectal examination may be necessary to identify them.

Endometriosis has been staged in a number of different ways. The American Society for Reproductive Medicine (ASRM) classification is designed to suggest prognosis in the management of subfertility. It scores adhesive damage and endometriomas highly but peritoneal disease scores low. There is poor correlation between ASRM score and levels of pain. Other authors have suggested that an accurate description of the type of endometriosis present and its location is a better description of the severity of the disease.

Transvaginal ultrasound scan is a cheap, safe and usually well-tolerated investigation. It is very effective at diagnosing endometriomas and possibly adenomyosis, but cannot reliably detect peritoneal disease.

MRI is also a reliable (though much more expensive) way to detect endometriomas. It is effective in the detection of adenomyosis and may also be helpful in the identification of bowel involvement preoperatively.[6]

A detailed history combined with a careful pelvic examination looking for nodules, fixity, pelvic masses and focal tenderness, followed by a therapeutic trial of hormones may allow the clinician to offer the woman a confident diagnosis with effective treatment without the need for a diagnostic laparoscopy.[5]

Treatment

The choice of treatment for any particular woman depends very considerably on her plans with regard to fertility or contraception and her personal preferences regarding the use of hormones and other drugs. Many women simply want to understand the nature of their symptoms and what the future may hold. The role of the clinician is then to provide her with the information she needs to make her own choices regarding future management. The opportunity to read facts and opinions for herself may be useful and a number of excellent websites exist for this purpose.[7,8]

MANAGEMENT OF SUBFERTILITY-ASSOCIATED ENDOMETRIOSIS

If a woman is trying to conceive she clearly cannot take any hormonal treatment. There is no improvement in fertility following a course of hormonal treatment.[9] However, simple analgesia is still appropriate, particularly during menstruation. The role of surgical treatment for stage III and IV disease is uncertain particularly given that in vitro fertilization (IVF) may be a very effective treatment. In the absence of pain it may be better to limit surgical treatment and consequently risks, in favour of proceeding straight to IVF. Endometriomas should be removed prior to IVF. Guidelines suggest that mild to minimal endometriosis should be treated at the time of laparoscopy if the woman is trying to conceive.

SIMPLE ANALGESIA

NSAIDs are effective in the control of pain related to endometriosis but no particular drug can be recommended.[10] Starting treatment 24 hours before the onset of pain can bring additional effectiveness. Paracetamol is also useful, perhaps combined with a stronger analgesic such as codeine. Moving on to stronger opiates should probably only be initiated by pain specialists. Adjuvant analgesics such as amitriptyline can be helpful (see Chapter 9).

CONTRACEPTIVES WHICH MAY BE EFFECTIVE AGAINST ENDOMETRIOSIS

Combined oral contraceptive pill

No particular combined oral contraceptive pill can be recommended over another, but they are helpful in reducing pelvic pain and dysmenorrhoea associated with endometriosis.[11] Contraindications to their use should be ruled out such as history of thrombosis or smoking in an older woman. Additional benefit may be derived from running several packets together (the so-called tricycle regime), particularly if symptoms are predominantly menstrual.

Progesterone-only oral contraception

As many women will become amenorrhoeic taking a progesterone-only pill (such as Cerazette® in the UK), this can be an option for women unable to take oestrogen.

Levonorgestrel – Secreting intrauterine system (LNG – IUS)

Although it has no licence for the management of endometriosis, because it induces amenorrhoea or minimal bleeding in a high proportion of women, the LNG – IUS can be very effective in the management of endometriosis-related pain[12] even for women who have not had children. Women should be warned about the likelihood of irregular bleeding and consequently pain for the first few months following insertion. Women with endometriosis often have greater than average pain during insertion and a light general anaesthetic may be appropriate for the procedure. Generic devices will be available in the near future and smaller devices are being developed.

Depo-Provera® and Nexplanon®

Although the rate of irregular bleeding is higher than that associated with the LNG – IUS, depot progestogen formulations such as

Depo-Provera® or Nexplanon®, when combined with the need for excellent contraception, may be an acceptable choice.

HORMONES TO INDUCE AMENORRHOEA

Although there are a number of treatments licensed and effective for the treatment of endometriosis, they all suppress rather than eradicate the disease. When treatment is stopped, endometriosis may well return and women should be aware of this from the outset. All three drugs suggested here are thought to be equally effective and a woman's choice is likely to depend on expected side-effect profile, mode of delivery and previous experience.

GnRH analogue

By suppressing the hypothalamic–pituitary axis, these drugs (goserelin, triptorelin and leuprorelin) reduce the level of circulating oestrogen which is thought to lead to atrophy of the endometrioid tissue. They have significant side effects which are essentially those of the menopause: hot flushes, depressed mood, skin changes, reduced libido, etc. Women should be warned that when starting a course, they may initially experience a worsening of their symptoms, often in association with the next and final period (the so-called 'flare effect'). Amenorrhoea and a steady reduction in symptoms over the next 2–3 months are then expected.

An important consequence of the use of GnRH analogue is loss of bone density which may be up to 10% in 6 months. Although it is not licensed for use beyond 6 months, GnRH analogue can be used with hormone replacement therapy (HRT) to prevent bone loss and reduce side effects. The HRT could be any continuous combined formulation although the only product licensed in the UK for this indication is tibolone. This combination of treatment has been shown to maintain quality of life and bone density for two years.[13] Anecdotal evidence suggests similar benefit for 10 years.[14] Women need to balance the benefit they are experiencing against the unknown risk of this regime.

High-dose progestogen

Medroxyprogesterone acetate (20–30 mg twice a day) or norethisterone (5 mg three times a day) can be used to suppress menstruation and are effective in the treatment of pain associated with endometriosis.[15] Decidualization of endometriotic deposits is induced. Irregular bleeding will reduce effective pain control and if this occurs, consideration should be given to increasing the dose to achieve amenorrhoea. Expected progesterone-related side effects include weight gain, tearfulness, bloating, skin changes and breast tenderness. Although women may be put off by an expected state of permanent premenstrual tension (PMT), some patients experience a sense of well-being. Delivered in tablet form, this treatment may be more acceptable to women than an injection which they cannot stop immediately.

Danazol

Although it is as effective as the first two treatments[16], danazol has a poor side-effect profile, including, rarely, irreversible voice deepening. Other side effects reflect its androgenic nature and include hair growth, weight gain, acne and cliteromegaly. For this reason it tends to be kept in reserve, but when other options are limited, it may have a useful place.

NEW THERAPEUTIC OPTIONS

Aromatase inhibitors have been used alone or in combination with standard endometriosis drugs. Although promising, this novel treatment has not yet been widely adopted.[17]

SURGICAL OPTIONS

Laparoscopic ablation

Various forms of energy have been used to ablate or excise peritoneal endometriosis, including electrical or laser cautery. The form of energy does not seem to matter, but surgical treatment would seem to be as effective as hormonal treatment.[18] Where more solid or fibrous elements of endometriosis are present, such as endometriomas or nodules, surgery may be required to achieve good symptom control, as hormonal treatment will only suppress the glandular component of the disease. Endometriomas are better treated by excision than by drainage and ablation alone. Given the high prevalence of endometriosis, the majority of treatments for peritoneal and mild adhesive disease can and should be performed by most gynaecologists ideally at the time of laparoscopic diagnosis. Where disease is extensive or frequently recurring, consideration should be given to referral of the patient to a centre with extensive experience in the surgical management of endometriosis.

Patients should be made aware of the risks of surgery, particularly when disease is extensive and involving the bowel.[19] Patients should also be aware that endometriosis is a recurrent disease and that the possibility of recurrence remains even after extensive laparoscopic surgery.[20] Some have put this as high as 50%, which is similar to the recurrence rate following hormonal treatment.

The ovarian reserve of women with severe endometriosis may be gradually eroded by repeated endometriomas formation and surgery to the ovary. Every effort should be made to preserve ovarian tissue if at all possible. The potential effect on fertility of endometriosis of whatever severity should always be discussed when a diagnosis is made, to allow the patient to discuss the issues and to make whatever choices are right for her, even when she has no immediate plans to conceive. If extensive surgery is planned and pregnancy is to be delayed, a discussion about the possibility of egg or embryo freezing, and its pros and cons may be helpful. This option may become more widespread in future as the success of such interventions improves. The opportunity to discuss such questions may be another reason to consider referral to a specialist centre before embarking on major surgery.

In women wishing to delay conception, consideration should be given to starting the combined oral contraceptive following surgery.[21]

Hysterectomy with bilateral salpingo-oophorectomy

If a woman's family is complete or if she has no wish to retain her fertility, removal of the ovaries may offer the most effective solution for her. The uterus is usually also removed to simplify hormone replacement. Removal of the uterus alone as a treatment for endometrioisis is illogical since it is an oestrogen-dependent disease and is driven by the ovaries. However, many women report symptom relief following removal of the uterus alone, although the mechanism for this is unclear. Retention of the uterus alone for use with the woman's own or donated eggs would be a possibility. At the time of surgery it is also important to try to treat any residual disease within the pelvis. Oestrogen replacement therapy should be given until the average age of the menopause, namely about 50–52 years. If extensive residual endometriosis is present, it may be sensible to give continuous combined HRT, to reduce the risk of stimulation and even malignant transformation in residual endometriotic deposits.[22]

Conclusion

Endometriosis is a common and debilitating disease. It can be extremely disruptive both in terms of symptoms and the pain of subfertility, leading to time off work and personal distress. Doctors must have adequate knowledge to recognise the significance and importance of pain symptoms and to offer women helpful information enabling them to make the right choices for their particular circumstances.

References

1. Eskenazi B, Warner ML. Epidemiology of endometriosis. *Obstet Gynecol Clin North Am* 1997;24:235–58.
2. Bulun SE. Endometriosis. *N Engl J Med* 2009;360:268–79.
3. Ozkan S, Murk W, Arici A. Endometriosis and infertility: epidemiology and evidence-based treatments. *Ann NY Acad Sci* 2008;1127:92–100.
4. Chapron C, Querleu D, Bruhat MA, Madelenat P, Fernandez H, Pierre F, Dubuisson JB. Surgical complications of diagnostic and operative gynaecological laparoscopy: a series of 29,966 cases. *Human Reprod* 1998;13:867–72.
5. Royal College of Obstetricians and Gynaecologists. *The Investigation and Management of Endometriosis*. Green-top Guideline No. 24. London: RCOG; 2006.
6. Dueholm M, Lundorf E. Transvaginal ultrasound or MRI for the diagnosis of adenomyosis. *Curr Opin Obstet Gynecol* 2007;19:505–12.
7. www.endometriosis-uk.org
8. www.nhs.uk/conditions/endometriosis/Pages/Introduction.aspx.
9. Hughes E, Brown J, Collins JJ, Farquhar C, Fedorkow DM, Vandekerckhove P. Ovulation suppression for endometriosis. *Cochrane Database Syst Rev* 2007;(3):CD000155.
10. Allen C, Hopewell S, Prentice A, Gregory D. Nonsteroidal anti-inflammatory drugs for pain in women with endometriosis. *Cochrane Database Syst Rev* 2009;(2):CD004753.
11. Davis L, Kennedy S, Moore J, Prentice A. Modern combined contraceptives for pain associated with endometriosis. *Cochrane Database Syst Rev* 2007;(3): CD001019.
12. Lockat FB, Emembolu JO, Konje JC. The efficacy, side-effects and continuation rates in women with symptomatic endometriosis undergoing treatment with an intra-uterine administered progestogen (levonorgestrel): a 3 year follow-up. *Human Reprod* 2005;20:789–93.
13. Sagsveen M, Farmer JE, Prentice A, Breeze A. Gonadotrophin-releasing hormone analogues for endometriosis: bone mineral density. *Cochrane Database Syst Rev* 2003;(4):CD001297.
14. Bedaiwy MA, Casper RF. Treatment with leuprolide acetate and hormonal add-back for up to 10 years in stage IV endometriosis patients with chronic pelvic pain. *Fertil Steril* 2006;86(1):220–2.
15. Prentice A, Deary AJ, Bland E. Progestagens and anti-progestagens for pain associated with endometriosis. *Cochrane Database Syst Rev* 2000;(2):CD002122.
16. Selak V, Farquhar C, Prentice A, Singla A. Danazol for pelvic pain associated with endometriosis. *Cochrane Database Syst Rev* 2007;(4): CD000068.

17. Bedaiwy MA, Mousa NA, Casper RF. Aromatase inhibitors: potential reproductive implications. *J Minim Invasive Gynecol* 2009;16:533–9.
18. Jacobson TZ, Duffy JM, Barlow D, Koninckx PR, Garry R. Laparoscopic surgery for pelvic pain associated with endometriosis. *Cochrane Database Syst Rev* 2009;(4):CD001300.
19. Slack A, Child T, Lindsey I, et al. Urological and colorectal complications following surgery for rectovaginal endometriosis. BJOG 2007;114:1278–82.
20. Abbott JA, Hawe J, Clayton RD, Garry R. The effects and effectiveness of laparoscopic excision of endometriosis: a prospective study with 2–5 year follow-up. *Human Reprod* 2003;(9):1922–7.
21. Vercellini P, Somigliana E, Viganò P, De Matteis S, Barbara G, Fedele L. Post-operative endometriosis recurrence: a plea for prevention based on pathogenic, epidemiological and clinical evidence. *Reprod Biomed Online.* 2010 Aug;21(2):259–65.
22. Al Kadri H, Hassan S, Al-Fozan HM, Hajeer A. Hormone therapy for endometriosis and surgical menopause. *Cochrane Database Syst Rev* 2009;(1): CD005997.

Further reading

Giudice LC. Endometriosis. *N Engl J Med* 2010;362:2389–98.

Kennedy S, Bergqvist A, Chapron C, et al. ESHRE guideline for the diagnosis and treatment of endometriosis. *Human Reprod* 2005;20:2698–704.

Revised American Society for Reproductive Medicine classification of endometriosis: 1996. *Fertil Steril* 1997;67:817–21.

9 Chronic pelvic pain

Chronic pelvic pain (CPP) may profoundly affect women's ability to function normally in their various roles. Repeated episodes of absence may lead to disruption of working life. Chronic pain may damage their ability to care for their children or maintain social networks, leading to relationship breakdown and loss of quality of life. Although some women have intractable pain, this chapter attempts to describe a variety of simple and effective interventions, which will improve quality of life for a large proportion of sufferers.

Definitions and epidemiology

Pain is defined by the International Association for the Study of Pain as an unpleasant sensory and emotional experience associated with actual or potential tissue damage, or described in such terms.[1] It is always subjective.

CPP can be defined in a number of ways, but perhaps the most useful is a symptom-based definition: intermittent or constant pain felt in the lower abdomen or pelvis, not associated exclusively with menstruation or intercourse and not associated with pregnancy or malignancy.

Definitions which rely on causality such as 'pelvic pain with no organic cause' are flawed because understanding of the causes of pelvic pain is imperfect. Measures of severity reliant on patients' behaviour – for example 'pain severe enough to disrupt work' – are also clearly affected by much more than the pain itself. An awareness of the definition used is an important factor in interpreting the literature and opinion on this subject.

CPP affects approximately 1 in 6 of the population.[2] Not all of these women will consult their GP and many will be managed appropriately in primary care. Women present to their GPs with CPP about as frequently as patients with back pain or asthma.[3]

Contributory factors in the genesis of CPP

Pelvic pain may arise from any structure in or related to the pelvis. Often there is more than one factor contributing to the pain. Assessment of the pain should seek to identify contributory factors rather than a single cause. Along with other pain syndromes, the function or dysfunction of the central nervous system in response to local factors is increasingly seen as crucial. Box 9.1 provides a list of possible contributory factors.

BOX 9.1 CONTRIBUTORY FACTORS IN THE GENESIS OF CHRONIC PELVIC PAIN

Gynaecological:

- Endometriosis
- Adenomyosis
- Adhesions
- Chronic pelvic inflammatory disease (PID)

Bowel-related:

- Irritable bowel syndrome
- Constipation

Bladder-related:

- Interstitial cystitis

Musculoskeletal:

- Symphisis pubis/sacroiliacs
- Abdominal or pelvic trigger points

Neurological:

- Nerve entrapment
- Neuropathic pain
- Central nervous system response to chronic pain

Psychological:

- Sleep disturbance, depression
- Physical, emotional or sexual abuse, past or current
- Specific health beliefs and concerns

CENTRAL NERVOUS SYSTEM FACTORS

Pain must be processed in the brain in order to be perceived. Factors such as depression and sleep disturbance might reasonably be expected to affect the pain experience but it is increasingly apparent that other factors within the central nervous system will also modify the experience of chronic pain.

At a local level, inflammatory mediators may recruit otherwise silent afferents or alter receptor function, possibly magnifying the pain signal. Within the spinal cord, activation within the dorsal horn is seen in response to a repeating signal from the periphery. This may result in magnification or modification of signals not only in that spinal segment, but also in two or three segments on either side of the original stimulus.

At any level in the spinal cord, information is received from a number of sources both somatic and visceral. Modification of the nerve pathways at this level may affect not only the original source but also inputs and outputs affecting other areas reporting to the same segment. For example, sensory input from bowel and bladder might be altered in a spinal segment, which is also receiving pain signals from the uterus. This 'scrambling' of information may also affect motor signals. It has been termed 'cross talk' or 'viscero-visceral mapping' and may explain the observation that irritable bowel syndrome is more common among women suffering from endometriosis than in the general population.

Within the spinal segment, inputs from one area may be 'rerouted' and interpreted by the brain as coming from another area mapping onto the same segment. For example, the uterus is innervated by T12-L2 which also innervates the skin area from above the symphysis and onto the anterior thighs. Pain from the uterus may therefore be perceived as coming from the abdominal wall and thighs. Sensation in these areas may even be affected. This has been termed referred pain or 'viscero-somatic mapping'.

The central nervous system is clearly a plastic system affected by numerous factors. In the presence of a repeated pain signal, changes which may promote, inhibit or modify the pain signal can occur at local, spinal and central levels. See Baranowski[4] for a review of CNS involvement in the genesis of pelvic pain.

GYNAECOLOGICAL FACTORS

Endometriosis

This disease is considered in much more detail in Chapter 8, but without doubt it may be a contributory factor in the generation of pelvic pain.

It is known that the extent of the disease seen laparoscopically correlates poorly with the degree of pain experienced. This may be partly due to other contributory factors such as depression or irritable bowel syndrome, but may also reflect our poor understanding of the factors which generate the pain of endometriosis. Endometriosis causes fibrosis and distortion of tissues and this may be a potent cause of pain, either directly or as a result of traction on nerves. It also releases a number of chemical mediators which themselves generate pain, stimulating or changing the behaviour of receptors and peripheral nerves.

The hallmark of endometriosis-related pain is its cyclical variation. Pain is characteristically cramping or aching in nature and felt suprapubically, but may be sharp or burning and radiate into the back or thighs. It is usually at its worst during menstruation (dysmenorrhoea), but builds up in the week or 10 days before the period. There may also be a peak at the time of ovulation. As it becomes more severe it may come to affect the whole month, but it retains its cyclical variation. It may be associated with dyspareunia (pain with intercourse) and dyschezia (pain on opening the bowels). It is important to enquire specifically about these symptoms.

Adenomyosis

A variant of endometriosis, adenomyosis describes endometrioid tissue within the myometrium. Like endometriosis, the pain is characteristically cyclical and may be associated with menstrual disruption.[5] It is not visible at laparoscopy but may be detected using MRI or ultrasound. These investigations are user dependent and published sensitivities and specificities may not be achieved outside centres of excellence.

Adhesions

Arising from previous surgery, infection or secondary to an inflammatory process such as endometriosis, adhesions are a common finding at laparoscopy but are not necessarily associated with pain. It may be that, when pain is present, the cause of the adhesions has also led to nerve damage and it is this which maintains the pain. Studies designed to assess the effect of adhesiolysis on pain are inconclusive either because they consider techniques which are not used in modern practice[6] or because of poor study design.[7]

PID

An acute upper genital tract infection with a STI is an important cause of pelvic pain and an important condition to detect in order to prevent damage to future fertility and onward transmission. This has been termed acute PID and may lead to damage such as adhesion formation or perhaps nerve damage leading to CPP. This combination of signs and symptoms has sometimes been labelled chronic PID.

Clearly, a pelvic infection might be recurrent (perhaps from poor treatment of a sexual partner). The common practice of treating women presenting with recurrent episodes of pelvic pain with antibiotics in order to be sure such an infection is not missed may be justifiable. However many women presenting in this way do not have active infection and once this has been ruled out using swabs and poor response to antibiotics, it is important that the true cause or contributory factors to her pain should be sought and treated.

Thought should be given to the social consequences of an incorrect diagnosis of an STI. It may also be that the episode of PID has left her with particular fears or concerns either about the circumstances surrounding the acquisition of the infection or its effects on her future fertility.

For a fuller discussion of the management of PID, see RCOG Green-top Guideline No. 32.[8]

BOWEL-RELATED FACTORS

Irritable bowel syndrome

Irritable bowel syndrome is common, affecting about 20% of the population, and may be diagnosed using the Rome criteria.[9] The important feature is whether the pain varies with changing bowel habit.

Constipation

This is common and although perhaps not usually the sole cause of CPP may well be an important contributory factor.

BLADDER-RELATED FACTORS

Interstitial cystitis

This is a poorly characterized inflammatory condition of the bladder wall which may be associated with pain and irritative bladder symptoms such as dysuria and frequency – for a review see Forrest and Dell.[10] Again the important question is whether the pain varies with bladder symptoms.

MUSCULOSKELETAL FACTORS

Bones and joints

Symphisis pubis dysfunction is a well-recognized cause of pain in pregnancy and may lead to longer-term pain and disability. The sacroiliac joints and lower spine may also be a cause of pain, which may be referred into the iliac fossae. Pain characteristically varies with movement or particular postures and gets worse over the course of the day. There is often some mild variation across the menstrual cycle as there is with arthritis. A physiotherapy assessment may be very helpful.

Trigger points

In recent years there has been increasing medical interest in the concept of trigger points. These are painful spots in the muscles of the body wall thought to result from chronically contracted and shortened muscles. Such chronic shortening might result from factors such as distortion of the bony pelvis or repeated adoption of a particular posture, perhaps as a result of pain. Trigger points have been identified in the abdominal wall and the pelvic floor, and various interventions have been tried such as botulinum toxin injections, acupuncture or physiotherapy. For a review, see Montenegro et al.[11]

NEUROLOGICAL FACTORS

Nerve entrapment

Nerves may become caught in the fibrous tissue associated with surgical scars, for example at the edge of a Pfannenstiel incision, the ilioinguinal and iliohypogastric nerves may become entrapped. Pain is characteristically stabbing, shooting or lancinating in nature, often associated with movement. A constant ache or a patch of numbness may also be present in the area of distribution of that nerve.

Neuropathic pain

If a nerve becomes damaged by a disease process such as endometriosis or adhesion formation, its function may be disrupted. Pain may result and this has been termed neuropathic pain. With increasing awareness of the effect of inflammatory mediators on nerve function, the concept that the function of the nerves themselves might be relevant and modifiable has been introduced into the management of CPP. The importance of the central nervous system's response to pain is discussed earlier in this chapter.

PSYCHOLOGICAL FACTORS

Psychological factors are bound to affect the pain experience and women are often ready to acknowledge that, when they are stressed, their pain is worse. This does not mean that the sources of worry are causing the pain. Depression and sleep disturbance should be specifically asked about and treated, but they are rarely the only relevant factor.

The link between abuse and pelvic pain is complex. It would seem however that if a woman has suffered abuse in the past, particularly if it is ongoing, she may be vulnerable to a chronic pain syndrome. If the abuse is of a sexual nature, this may be reflected in increased symptoms of pelvic pain.[12]

Initial assessment

HISTORY

Allowing the patient to tell her story is time well spent. The story of the onset of the pain, its variation with the cycle, the bowels, with movement, may well help to characterise its origins. A full sexual history is important. The words she uses and the connections she makes may give you clues about her health beliefs. The simple act of listening and taking her pain seriously may be therapeutic in itself.[13]

In women of reproductive age, pelvic pain alone is very rarely a presenting symptom of sinister pathology, but some red flag symptoms might warrant a more urgent approach. For example, abnormal vaginal bleeding, particularly postcoital, might herald cervical carcinoma. Weight loss, new bowel symptoms over the age of 40, or a family history might warrant further investigation for bowel or ovarian cancer. Persistent haematuria should prompt cytology of the urine.

EXAMINATION

The abdomen should be examined looking particularly for tenderness. Trigger points, highly localized tender spots, may be apparent in the abdominal wall. A vaginal examination should be performed, possibly including swabs for STI. The size and tenderness of the uterus and any adnexal tenderness should be noted. The fornices should be carefully examined looking for focal tenderness which might suggest nodular endometriosis. Trigger points in the pelvic floor may also be identified. The woman's behaviour during the examination may give clues to anxieties or concerns she may have. The vaginal examination might reasonably be deferred if there is not enough time to explore any feelings which it provokes.

INVESTIGATIONS

Swabs for STIs should be taken if appropriate from the sexual history, even if no other symptoms of PID are present. Further investigations should be directed by associated symptoms. An ultrasound scan is often helpful particularly to address specific health concerns that the woman may have, for example 'Might this be ovarian cancer?' An MRI scan can be helpful to assess the possibility of adenomyosis.

Diagnostic laparoscopy may be useful particularly if the woman is concerned about fertility. However, since a negative laparoscopy does not rule out an endometriosis-like condition as a cause of pain, it may be more useful to embark on a therapeutic trial of hormones if the history is suggestive of endometriosis rather than automatically perform a diagnostic laparoscopy.

Management

The woman will no doubt have thought about her pain and may have developed quite clear views about what might be causing it and how it should be investigated and treated. Uncovering these health beliefs and addressing specific concerns is an essential part of the management of CPP. Women often seek help for their pain because they want an explanation. This may not always be possible, but addressing specific concerns, ruling these out as a cause of pain and then providing a plausible explanation may be acceptable.

The aim of treatment should be to allow the woman to return to as near normal function as possible. Whilst an acceptable level of pain control is obviously important, it may be helpful to actively focus on the goals she wants to achieve and reduce the focus on pain as such.

If symptoms are not readily resolved with initial management, a multidisciplinary approach to treatment has been shown to be helpful.[14] This may involve physiotherapy, psychological and pain management experts as well as gynaecologists. There is limited evidence to recommend any particular treatment in the absence of a specific diagnosis.[15] If an adequate programme has been established, allowing the patient to return to a good level of function, the aim should be to return the patient's management to primary care accessing secondary care only if new problems arise.

Management will also depend on her fertility aspirations and whether or not she wants or needs contraception. It may involve a number of strategies to address the various identified components of the pain. For example if it is thought that irritable bowel syndrome is a component of the pain, dietary modification by the patient to identify particular foods which provoke pain may be helpful. Mebeverine, a smooth muscle relaxant, may give some relief.

The management of endometriosis is discussed in Chapter 8. All strongly cyclical pain may benefit from the hormonal regimes used in the management of endometriosis, even if a specific diagnosis of endometriosis or adenomyosis has not been made.

MANAGING THE PAIN EMPIRICALLY

NSAIDs

None of the routinely available NSAIDs is more effective than the others in treating pain, although individuals may prefer one to another.[16] Rotating from one to another may be helpful. They should be taken regularly rather than intermittently when the pain is bad to exploit the anti-inflammatory action. Rectal diclofenac may be useful during peaks of pain.

Paracetamol

Regular paracetamol is effective and should be used if necessary with other analgesics.

Codeine

Drugs such as codeine may be helpful in managing peaks of pain such as during menstruation, although side effects often limit their use. Prescription of morphine-like drugs is an important line to cross in the management of benign pain and should probably only be undertaken by specialists in the field after exclusion of other options.

Adjuvant analgesics

Particularly when pain sounds neuropathic in nature (for example, lancinating, burning or shooting), amitriptyline (25 mg increasing if necessary to a maximum of 150 mg, usually 50–75 mg, although some patients tolerate 10–20 mg better) or gabapentin (300–600 mg three times a day) may be useful. They can be very effective and often allow other analgesics to be reduced.

Surgical approaches

LUNA has been demonstrated to be ineffective and should not be used in the management of CPP.[17] Presacral neurectomy may be effective although more research is needed to establish its risk–benefit profile.

Hysterectomy and removal of the ovaries without addressing the components of pain is unlikely to be helpful unless the pain is strongly cyclical. A trial of GnRH analogue may be helpful to assess the effect of ovarian suppression before taking the decision to offer hysterectomy.

Complementary therapies

Although little evidence of benefit exists in defence of these treatments, many women find them extremely helpful and if function is the touchstone, women should be encouraged to try them if they wish.

Conclusion

Pelvic pain is common and extremely disruptive, not only to the patient herself but also to those dependent on her. Early intervention, taking her concerns seriously and providing effective diagnosis and management may prevent the secondary consequences of chronic pain both social and neurological and allow return to satisfactory function. Simple assessment often from the patient history alone can identify therapeutic opportunities which, even if the pain cannot be eliminated, may reduce the overall pain burden.

References

1. International Association for the Study of Pain. *Pain Terms: A Current List with Definitions and Notes on Usage*. Seattle: IASP; 2011 [www.iasp-pain.org/AM/Template.cfm?Section=Pain_Defi. . .isplay.cfm&ContentID=1728].
2. Zondervan KT, Yudkin PL, Vessey MP, et al. The community prevalence of chronic pelvic pain in women and associated illness behaviour. *Br J Gen Pract* 2001;51:541–7.
3. Zondervan KT, Yudkin PL, Vessey MP, Dawes MG, Barlow DH, Kennedy SH. Prevalence and incidence of chronic pelvic pain in primary care:

evidence from a national general practice database. *Br J Obstet Gynaecol* 1999;106:1149–55.
4. Baranowski AP. Chronic pelvic pain. *Best Pract Res Clin Gastroenterol* 2009; 23:593–610.
5. Mehasseb MK, Habiba MA. Adenomyosis uteri: an update. *The Obstetrician & Gynaecologist* 2009;11:41–47.
6. Peters AA, Trimbos-Kemper GC, Admiraal C, Trimbos JB, Hermans J. A randomized clinical trial on the benefit of adhesiolysis in patients with intraperitoneal adhesions and chronic pelvic pain. *Br J Obstet Gynaecol* 1992;99,59–62.
7. Swank DJ, Swank-Bordewijk SC, Hop WC, et al. Laparoscopic adhesiolysis in patients with chronic abdominal pain: a blinded randomised controlled multi-centre trial. *Lancet* 2003;361:1247–51.
8. Royal College of Obstetricians and Gynaecologists. *Management of Acute Pelvic Inflammatory Disease*. Green-top Guideline No. 32. London: RCOG; 2009.
9. Drossman DA, Dumitrascu DL. Rome III: New standard for functional gastrointestinal disorders. *J Gastrointestin Liver Dis* 2006;15:237–41.
10. Forrest JB, Dell JR. Successful management of interstitial cystitis in clinical practice. *Urology* 2007;69:82–6.
11. Montenegro ML, Vasconcelos EC, Candido Dos Reis FJ, Noqueira AA, Poli-Neto OB. Physical therapy in the management of women with chronic pelvic pain. *Int J Clin Pract* 2008;62:263–269.
12. Lampe A, Doering S, Rumpold G, et al. Chronic pain syndromes and their relation to childhood abuse and stressful life events. *J Psychosom Res* 2003;54:361–7.
13. Price J, Farmer G, Harris J, Hope T, Kennedy S, Mayou R. Attitudes of women with chronic pelvic pain to the gynaecological consultation: a qualitative study. *BJOG* 2006;113:446–452.
14. Peters AA, van Dorst E, Jellis B, van Zuuren E, Hermans J, Trimbos JB. A randomized clinical trial to compare two different approaches in women with chronic pelvic pain. *Obstet Gynecol* 1991;77:740–4.
15. Stones W, Cheong YC, Howard FM. Interventions for treating chronic pelvic pain in women. *Cochrane Database Syst Rev* 2005;(2): CD000387.
16. Marjoribanks J, Proctor M, Farquhar C, Derks RS. Nonsteroidal anti-inflammatory drugs for dysmenorrhoea. *Cochrane Database Syst Rev* 2010; (1):CD001751.
17. National Institute for Health and Clinical Excellence. *LUNA for Chronic Pelvic Pain*. Interventional Procedure Guidance 234. London: NICE; 2008

Further reading and other resources

The International Pelvic Pain Society [www.pelvicpain.org/]
The Gut Trust website [www.theibsnetwork.org/]
The Cystitis and Overactive Bladder Foundation [www.cobfoundation.org/]

Allen C, Hopewell S, Prentice A. Nonsteroidal anti-inflammatory drugs for pain in women with endometriosis. *Cochrane Database Syst Rev* 2005;(4): CD004753.
Cheong Y, Stones W. Chronic pelvic pain: aetiology and therapy. *Best Pract Res Clin Obstet Gynaecol* 2006;20:695–711.
Royal College of Obstetricians and Gynaecologists. *The Initial Management of Chronic Pelvic Pain*. Green-top Guideline No. 41. London: RCOG; 2005.
Vercellini P, Somigliana E, Vigano P, Abbiati A, Barbara G, Fedele L. Chronic pelvic pain in women: etiology, pathogenesis and diagnostic approach. *Gynecol Endocrinol* 2009; 25:149–158.
Vercellini P, Vigano P, Somigliana E, Abbiati A, Barbara G, Fedele L. Medical, surgical and alternative treatments for chronic pelvic pain in women: a descriptive review. *Gynecol Endocrinol* 2009;25:208–21.
Wiffen P, Collins S, McQuay H, Carroll D, Jadad A, Moore A. Anticonvulsant drugs for acute and chronic pain. *Cochrane Database Syst Rev* 2000;(3): CD001133.

10 Delayed menarche

In the absence of endocrine or systemic disease or drug therapy, and in the presence of a normal chromosome complement, women require a functioning hypothalamic–pituitary–ovarian axis – with a responding endometrium and genital outflow tract – to menstruate.

In developed countries the menarche occurs between the ages of 10 and 16 in most girls.[1] The first cycles tend to be anovular, there is wide variation in cycle length, and the menstruations are usually pain-free and occur without warning. By 6 years after the menarche 80% of cycles are ovulatory, with the number reaching over 95% by 12 years.

There has been a secular trend to earlier menarche over the past century with a decrease of about 3 to 4 months per decade in industrialised areas such as Europe, US and Japan. Thus the average age of menarche in 1840 was 16.5, and now averages 13.

The reasons for the fall of menarcheal age are unclear but one interpretation is that it reflects improvement in health and environmental conditions.[2,3] It now appears that this trend is levelling off in many countries such as Britain, Iceland, Italy, Poland and Sweden. Indeed, there appears now to be a reversal of the fall with a gradual increase in the age of menarche in Britain since the birth cohort of 1945. However in other countries, the fall in age is still continuing.

Factors affecting the age of menarche

The age of menarche is determined by a combination of factors which include genetic influences, socio-economic conditions, general health and wellbeing, nutritional status, certain types of exercise, and family size. The importance of genetic factors is illustrated by the similar age of menarche in members of an ethnic population and in mother–daughter pairs. Similarly, twin studies have shown a closer relationship in menarcheal age in identical (3 months) than in non-identical twins (12 months). Social class differences are disappearing in many countries. It is well known that delayed menarche is a feature of chronic disease.

BODY WEIGHT AND FAT

The role of birth weight and proportion of body fat in menarcheal age has received considerable attention.[3] It is well known that anorexia and malnutrition are associated with delayed menarche, and both conditions can induce secondary amenorrhoea. A regular menstrual cycle will not occur if the body mass index (BMI) is less than $19 kg/m^2$. Fat appears to be critical to a normally functioning hypothalamic–pituitary–gonadal axis. It is estimated that at least 22% of body weight should be fat to maintain ovulatory cycles. The candidate mediator is the hormone leptin, secreted by fat cells and affecting pulsatility.

DIET

The composition of diet in childhood can also affect menarcheal age.[4] Girls who consume more (energy-adjusted) animal protein and less vegetable protein at ages 3 to 5 years have an earlier menarche. Conversely, a diet high in fibre is associated with a delayed menarche.

EXERCISE

Intense exercise such as athletics, gymnastics and ballet is associated with a delayed menarche.[5,6] It has been suggested that each year of premenarcheal training delays menarche by 5 months, but the mechanisms involved are not fully understood, although a more linear physique may make a difference. It is thought that a combination of biological selection and social factors affect menarche.

FAMILY SITUATION

Family size and birth order also influence age of menarche. There is a tendency to later menarche in girls from larger families and there is a tendency to precocity in girls born later in the family.[3,5] Again the mechanisms are unclear.

ENVIRONMENTAL/HORMONALLY ACTIVE CHEMICALS

The significance of early-life exposure to environmental or hormonally active chemicals is also a growing area of debate. In a follow-up of 594 children from the North Carolina Infant Feeding Study, born between 1978 and 1982, a slight (but not statistically significant) decrease in age at sexual maturation (defined using Tanner scores based on the acquisition of secondary sexual characteristics) was noted in girls exposed to higher transplacental levels of polychlorinated biphenyls or dichlorodiphenyl dichloroethene. In the same study, girls that were bottle-fed showed a tendency (non-significant) to mature later.[7] Accidental contamination of the Michigan food chain with polybrominated biphenyls led to the exposure of more than 4000 individuals in 1973. Breast-fed girls exposed to high levels of polybrominated biphenyls in utero had an earlier age at menarche (mean age = 11.6 years) than breast-fed girls exposed to lower levels in utero (mean age = 12.2–12.6 years) or girls who were not breast fed (mean age = 12.7 years).[8] These associations clearly need further investigation.

Investigating delayed menarche

How long should a general practitioner wait before investigating the girl who has never menstruated? Since most girls will have menstruated by the age of 16, this could be considered to be the upper age of the normal menarche.[9,10] However, referral is essential earlier if secondary sex characteristics have not developed or there appear to be anatomical disorders of the genital tract or signs of a chromosome abnormality. Rarer possibilities are Androgen Insensitivity Syndrome, previously known as testicular feminisation (maturation of breasts with absent axillary and pubic hair; absent uterus with normal or short vagina; 46XY with intra-abdominal testes) or Turner syndrome (many variants, but with typical short stature; sexual infantilism; webbing of the neck; cubitus valgus; 45XO with streak gonads). Absent development of the lower genital tract resulting in haematocolpos is another rare cause where secondary sexual development will be normal. There may be intermittent lower abdominal pain, a lower abdominal cystic swelling (confirmed on ultrasound) and a tense blue-coloured membrane may be seen at the introitus. Referral is obviously necessary for incision and drainage.

If secondary sexual development is normal or appears to be progressing satisfactorily, and there is no anatomical problem, then the likely cause is hormonal which can elucidated with an endocrine screen. Follow-up of women diagnosed with menstrual disorders in their teens is recommended.[11]

References

1. Gluckman PD, Hanson MA. Evolution, development and timing of puberty. *Trends Endocrinol Metab* 2006;17:7–12.
2. Parent AS, Teilmann G, Juul A, Skakkebaek NE, Toppari J, Bourguignon JP. The timing of normal puberty and the age limits of sexual precocity:

variations around the world, secular trends, and changes after migration. *Endocr Rev* 2003;24:668–93.
3. Mishra GD, Cooper R, Tom SE, Kuh D. Early life circumstances and their impact on menarche and menopause. *Womens Health (Lond Engl)* 2009;5:175–90.
4. Günther AL, Karaolis-Danckert N, Kroke A, Remer T, Buyken AE. Dietary protein intake throughout childhood is associated with the timing of puberty. *J Nutr* 2010;140:565–71.
5. Morris DH, Jones ME, Schoemaker MJ, Ashworth A, Swerdlow AJ. Determinants of age at menarche in the UK: analyses from the Breakthrough Generations Study. *Br J Cancer* 2010;103:1760–4.
6. Thein-Nissenbaum JM, Carr KE. Female athlete triad syndrome in the high school athlete. *Phys Ther Sport* 2011;12:108–16.
7. Gladen BC, Ragan NB, Rogan WJ. Pubertal growth and development and prenatal and lactational exposure to polychlorinated biphenyls and dichlorodiphenyl dichloroethene. *J Pediatr* 2000;136:490–6.
8. Blanck HM, Marcus M, Tolbert PE, et al. Age at menarche and tanner stage in girls exposed in utero and postnatally to polybrominated biphenyl. *Epidemiology* 2000;11:641–7.
9. Hickey M, Balen A. Menstrual disorders in adolescence: investigation and management. *Hum Reprod Update* 2003;9:493–504.
10. Peacock A, Alvi NS, Mushtaq T. Period problems: disorders of menstruation in adolescents. *Arch Dis Child* 2012;97:554–60.
11. Wiksten-Almströmer M, Hirschberg AL, Hagenfeldt K. Prospective follow-up of menstrual disorders in adolescence and prognostic factors. *Acta Obstet Gynecol Scand* 2008;87:1162–8.

11 Premature ovarian failure

Premature ovarian failure (POF) is a cessation in the normal functioning of the ovaries in a woman younger than age 40 years.[1,2] The condition is common. Overall, POF is responsible for 4%–18% of cases of secondary amenorrhoea and 10%–28% of primary amenorrhoea. It is estimated to affect 1% of women younger than 40 years and 0.1% of those under 30 years.[3] Early menopause refers to menopause that occurs at or before age 45 years.[4] Both POF and early menopause occur well below the median age of natural menopause (age 51 years in the UK).[5]

The terms premature ovarian failure and premature menopause are often used interchangeably, though there is debate about which term is best. Some women with POF will present with oligomenorrhoea and have persisting sporadic ovarian activity.[6] Menopause implies permanent cessation of ovarian activity and menstruation. Therefore, unless the woman has undergone bilateral oophorectomy, menstruation can recommence, albeit unpredictably and erratically, and spontaneous pregnancy may still occur.

Symptoms and health consequences of POF

The most common first symptom of POF is irregular periods. Others may present through infertility services or through investigation of primary amenorrhoea (see Chapter 10) or secondary amenorrhoea after ceasing either COCs or long-acting progestogens. Some women with POF also have symptoms of estrogen deficiency, similar to those of women with ovarian failure in their 50s. These may include:

- hot flushes and night sweats
- irritability, poor concentration
- decreased libido and dyspareunia
- vaginal dryness.

Premature ovarian failure is frequently associated with autoimmune disorders, particularly hypothyroidism (25%), Addison's disease (3%)

and diabetes mellitus (2.5%).[6] Premature ovarian failure frequently is associated with autoimmune disorders such as:

- hypothyroidism
- Addison's disease
- diabetes mellitus
- Crohn's disease
- vitiligo
- pernicious anaemia
- systemic lupus erythematosus
- rheumatoid arthritis.

Addison's disease may be present as part of a polyglandular failure syndrome. The type I syndrome is associated with POF. It comprises adrenal failure, hypoparathyroidism and chronic mucocutaneous candidiasis and mainly occurs in children. The type II syndrome may present much later with hypothyroidism and is less consistently associated with POF. It is important that autoimmune diseases should be screened for in women with primary POF.

Mean life expectancy in women with menopause before the age of 40 years is 2 years shorter than that in women with menopause after the age of 55 years.[4,7] Women with untreated premature menopause are at increased risk of developing osteoporosis, cardiovascular disease, dementia, cognitive decline and parkinsonism, but are at lower risk of breast malignancy. Premature menopause can lead to reduced peak bone mass (if the woman is younger than 25 years) or early bone loss thereafter.

Aetiology: primary POF

Primary POF can occur in women of any age, even below the age of 20. It can present as primary or secondary amenorrhoea. About 10%–20% of women with POF have a family history of the condition. While some cases of POF can be genetic, in the great majority of cases no cause can be found.

Traditional texts have distinguished between follicular depletion and dysfunction. In the absence of non-invasive tests to differentiate between the two, the only alternative is laparoscopic ovarian biopsy. However, validity of biopsies has been questioned, with pregnancies occurring despite lack of follicles on histological examination.

CHROMOSOME ABNORMALITIES

X chromosome

A critical region which relates to normal ovarian function has been identified on the X-chromosome (POF1), which ranges from Xq13 to Xq26.[8,9] A second gene of paternal origin (POF2) has also been identified, located at Xq13.3 to q21.1. Idiopathic POF can be familial or sporadic and the familial pattern of inheritance is compatible with X-linked (with incomplete penetrance) or an autosomal dominant mode of inheritance. In Turner syndrome, complete absence of one X chromosome (45XO) results in ovarian dysgenesis and primary ovarian failure but this may be incomplete due to mosaicism. There can then be some ovarian activity, usually short lived. Familial POF has been linked with fragile X permutations. Fragile X mutations occur at least ten times more often in women with POF than the general population. Therefore, as women with POF can become spontaneously pregnant they should be screened for fragile X.

Down syndrome

Women with Down syndrome (trisomy 21) also have an early menopause.

BEPS (benign edematous polysynovitis) syndrome

This is a rare autosomal dominant condition that leads to congenital abnormalities of the eye, including blepharophimosis, ptosis and epicanthus inversis. In BEPS I, eyelid malformation co-segregates with POF and has been mapped to chromosome 3q17.

Follicle-stimulating hormone receptor gene polymorphism and inhibin B mutation

Resistance to the action of gonadotrophins can lead to the clinical features of POF and this has been shown in a cohort of Finnish families. This is a very rare cause. In addition, a mutation in the inhibin gene that has a frequency ten-fold higher than in control women (7.0% versus 0.7%) has been identified.

ENZYME DEFICIENCIES

A number of enzyme deficiencies have been found to be associated with an increased risk of POF. The most common of these is the autosomal recessive condition of galactosaemia, in which there is a deficiency in the enzyme galactose-1-phosphate uridyltransferase. Other enzyme abnormalities associated with POF include deficiencies of 17α-hydroxylase, 17–20 desmolase and cholesterol desmolase. Deficiency of 17α-hydroxylase can prevent estradiol synthesis, which leads to primary amenorrhoea and elevated levels of gonadotrophins, even though developing follicles are present.

Women with a deficiency of cholesterol desmolase are not able to produce biologically active steroids and rarely survive to adulthood.

AUTOIMMUNE DISEASE

Circulating antiovarian antibodies have been found in 10%–69% of women with POF but also in a significant number of controls. Anti-gonadotrophin receptor antibodies have been isolated, but their significance remains unclear. Antibodies directed against steroid-producing cells have proved most promising in terms of predicting which women may develop ovarian failure as part of the polyglandular syndrome but these are found in a minority of those with POF.

Aetiology: secondary POF

Secondary POF is becoming more important as survival after the treatment of malignancy continues to improve.[10] At present there is no evidence that ovarian stimulation for assisted conception advances the age of menopause.[11] The causes of secondary POF are detailed below.

CHEMOTHERAPY AND RADIOTHERAPY

The likelihood of ovarian failure after chemotherapy or radiotherapy depends on the agent used, dosage levels, interval between treatments and, particularly, the age of the woman, which probably reflects the age-related progressive natural decline in the oocyte pool. The prepubertal ovary is more resistant to the effects of chemotherapeutic alkylating agents. However, suppression of menstruation with oral contraceptives or GnRH analogues in post-menarcheal women to conserve ovarian function has produced conflicting results.

Radiation-induced ovarian failure usually results in sterility when the total dose exceeds 6 Gy.[12] As with chemotherapy, however, prepubertal girls are more resistant to irradiation. While menstruation can resume after therapy, premature menopause can occur leading to a shorter reproductive life. Surgical transposition of the ovaries outside the direct field of treatment has been described. High-dose pelvic radiotherapy will have long-term effects on the uterus and its vasculature. Adverse pregnancy outcomes include an increased risk of early pregnancy loss, preterm birth and delivery of infants with low or very low birth weights.

BILATERAL OOPHORECTOMY

This results in an immediate menopause. The implications of this procedure require detailed preoperative discussion.

HYSTERECTOMY WITHOUT OOPHORECTOMY

This can induce ovarian failure.[13,14] The underlying aetiology is uncertain and may depend on ovarian function preceding hysterectomy. It is essential to counsel women about this preoperatively. The diagnosis may be difficult, as not all women have estrogen deficiency symptoms and, in the absence of a uterus, the pointer of amenorrhoea is absent. A case could be made for annual estimates of levels of follicle stimulating hormone (FSH) in women who have had a hysterectomy before the age of 40.[15]

UTERINE ARTERY EMBOLIZATION

This procedure can also lead to ovarian failure, but is extremely rare in women under 45 years of age. However, it is possible that a case can be made for annual FSH estimations in women who undergo this intervention before the age of 40.

INFECTION

Tuberculosis and mumps are infections that have been implicated most commonly. In most cases, normal ovarian function returns after infection with mumps. Malaria, varicella and shigella infections have also been implicated in POF.

Investigation

Investigations of premature menopause are:

- estimates of levels of FSH in serum (two samples taken 1 month apart)
- thyroid function tests

- autoimmune screen for polyendocrinopathy
- chromosome analysis and screening for fragile X, especially in women younger than 30 years
- estimates of bone mineral density through dual-energy X-ray (optional)
- adrenocorticotrophic hormone stimulation test if Addison's disease is suspected (optional).

The diagnostic usefulness of ovarian biopsy outside the context of a research setting has yet to be proved. Assessment of ovarian reserve is a controversial area. A number of ovarian reserve tests have been designed to determine oocyte reserve and quality. Parameters of ovarian reserve that have been studied include FSH, luteinising hormone (LH), estradiol, inhibin B, anti-Müllerian hormone, total antral follicle count and ovarian volume. Reviews of ovarian reserve tests has shown that they have only modest to poor predictive properties.[16–19]

POF, fertility and contraception

While women with POF are unlikely to become spontaneously pregnant, this can still occur due to spasmodic ovarian activity. Elevated FSH levels do not mean that a woman is infertile. The lifetime chance of spontaneous conception in women with karyotypically normal POF has been estimated at 5%–15%, with the age of the woman at the time of diagnosis being an important determinant. There is no proven treatment to improve a woman's ability to have a baby naturally. Donor oocyte IVF is the treatment of choice. Women with spontaneous, karyotypically normal POF have similar success rates to women who undergo conventional IVF. The age of the oocyte rather than the age of the recipient determines the chance of success. Oocyte donation also is an option for women with Turner syndrome and pregnancy rates in observational studies are similar to those with oocyte donation for other indications. The risk of miscarriage, however, is greater. Cardiovascular and other complications such as hypertension and pre-eclampsia occur more frequently in women with Turner syndrome.

In women having chemotherapy or radiotherapy, IVF with embryo freezing prior to treatment currently offers the highest likelihood of future pregnancy. However this depends on the woman having a partner with whom she wishes to have a family. While advances in oocyte preservation have improved live birth rates, this technique is still less successful than embryo freezing. Ovulation induction risks delaying treatment in those with aggressive tumours, and in women with hormone-sensitive tumours such as breast cancer there is the additional concern regarding the safety of ovarian stimulation. Cryopreservation of ovarian tissue is still largely experimental, although pregnancies have been reported. This technique would be an option for prepubertal girls where ovulation induction is not possible.

Because of the risk of spontaneous pregnancy, if the woman does not want to have (further) children she would need to consider continuing an effective form of contraception. The levonorgestrel-releasing IUCD would also provide the progestogen component of a HRT regimen. The next decision will be duration of contraception. Traditionally, women have been advised that contraception can be stopped if they have been amenorrhoeic for 2 years before the age of 50 years and 1 year above that. However, the menstrual pattern will be difficult to establish if she is using HRT or the levonorgestrel-releasing IUCD and she could be advised to continue with contraception until the age of 55 years.

Management

OESTROGEN REPLACEMENT THERAPY

Oestrogen replacement therapy is the mainstay of treatment for women with POF and is recommended until the average age of natural menopause which is about 51 in the UK. This view is endorsed by national and international regulatory bodies. There is no evidence that oestrogen replacement increases the risk of breast cancer to a level greater than that found in normally menstruating women and women with POF do not need to start mammographic screening early.[20] HRT or the combined oestrogen and progestogen contraceptive pill may be used.[1] The latter has the psychological benefit of being a treatment used by many of the woman's peer group and this is important when dealing with young women or teenagers. Women with POF who take HRT may need a higher dose of estrogen to control vasomotor symptoms than women in their 50s. Some women complain of reduced libido or sexual function despite apparently adequate doses of oestrogen replacement. Testosterone should be considered and a testosterone patch for female use is available.[21] Natural 17β-estradiol may be better for uterine development and possibly bone protection than synthetic oestrogens such as ethinyl estradiol as found in the COC. Natural 17β-estradiol is used to help facilitate uterine development prior to ovum donation.

No clinical trial evidence attests the efficacy or safety of the use of non-oestrogen-based treatments, such as bisphosphonates, strontium ranelate or raloxifene, in these women. Their effects on the developing fetal skeleton are unknown. Alternative and complementary therapies are of unknown benefit and their safety is unproven.

COUNSELLING

Women who suffer from or are at risk of developing POF must be provided with adequate information. Those undergoing chemoradiotherapy, hysterectomy, uterine artery embolization or oophorectomy before the age of 40 should be advised about POF and the health risks if untreated. POF is a difficult diagnosis to accept, especially if a woman wishes to have children.[22] National self-support groups for POF exist and these provide helpful psychological support for many women.

Conclusion

Premature and early ovarian failure are common. Untreated they are associated with an increased risk of osteoporosis, cardiovascular disease, dementia and parkinsonism. These women require HRT until the average of the natural menopause. The diagnosis can be devastating and these women need sensitive management preferably in dedicated clinical services.

References

1. Vujovic S, Brincat M, Erel T, et al.; European Menopause and Andropause Society. EMAS position statement: Managing women with premature ovarian failure. *Maturitas* 2010;67:91–3.
2. Map of Medicine Menopause [http://healthguides.mapofmedicine.com/choices/map/menopause1.html].
3. Coulam CB, Adamson SC, Annegers JF. Incidence of premature ovarian failure. *Obstet Gynecol* 1986;67:604–6.
4. Shuster LT, Rhodes DJ, Gostout BS, Grossardt BR, Rocca WA. Premature menopause or early menopause: long-term health consequences. *Maturitas* 2010;65:161–6.
5. Mishra G, Hardy R, Kuh D. Are the effects of risk factors for timing of menopause modified by age? Results from a British birth cohort study. *Menopause* 2007; 14: 717–24.
6. Nelson LM. Clinical practice. Primary ovarian insufficiency. *N Engl J Med* 2009;360:606–14.
7. Rocca WA, Grossardt BR, de Andrade M, Malkasian GD, Melton LJ. Survival patterns after oophorectomy in premenopausal women: a population-based cohort study. *Lancet Oncol* 2006;7:821–8.

8. The ESHRE Capri Workshop Group. Genetic aspects of female reproduction. *Hum Reprod Update* 2008;14:293–307.
9. Dixit H, Rao L, Padmalatha V, et al. Genes governing premature ovarian failure. *Reprod Biomed Online* 2010;20:724–40.
10. Basta NO, James PW, Gomez-Pozo B, Craft AW, McNally RJ. Survival from childhood cancer in northern England, 1968–2005. *Br J Cancer* 2011;105:1402–8.
11. Elder K, Mathews T, Kutner E, et al. Impact of gonadotrophin stimulation for assisted reproductive technology on ovarian ageing and menopause. *Reprod Biomed Online* 2008;16:611–6.
12. Wallace WH, Thomson AB, Saran F, Kelsey TW. Predicting age of ovarian failure after radiation to a field that includes the ovaries. *Int J Radiat Oncol Biol Phys* 2005;62:738–44.
13. Farquhar CM, Sadler L, Harvey SA, Stewart AW. The association of hysterectomy and menopause: a prospective cohort study. *BJOG* 2005;112:956–62.
14. Halmesmäki KH, Hurskainen RA, Cacciatore B, Tiitinen A, Paavonen JA. Effect of hysterectomy or LNG-IUS on serum inhibin B levels and ovarian blood flow. *Maturitas* 2007;57:279–85.
15. Hehenkamp WJ, Volkers NA, Broekmans FJ, et al. Loss of ovarian reserve after uterine artery embolization: a randomized comparison with hysterectomy. *Hum Reprod* 2007;22:1996–2005.
16. Lambalk CB, van Disseldorp J, de Koning CH, Broekmans FJ. Testing ovarian reserve to predict age at menopause. *Maturitas.* 2009;63:280–91.
17. Broekmans FJ, Kwee J, Hendriks DJ, Mol BW, Lambalk CB. A systematic review of tests predicting ovarian reserve and IVF outcome. *Hum Reprod Update* 2006;12:685–718.
18. Anderson RA, Nelson SM, Wallace WH. Measuring anti-Müllerian hormone for the assessment of ovarian reserve: When and for whom is it indicated? *Maturitas* 2012;71:28–33.
19. Faculty of Family Planning and Reproductive Health Care Clinical Effectiveness Unit. FFPRHC Guidance Contraception for women aged over 40 years. July 2010 [http://www.fsrh.org/pdfs/ContraceptionOver40July10.pdf].
20. Ewertz M, Mellemkjaer L, Poulsen AH, et al. Hormone use for menopausal symptoms and risk of breast cancer. A Danish cohort study. *Br J Cancer* 2005;92:1293–7.
21. Wylie K, Rees M, Hackett G, et al. Androgens, health and sexuality in women and men. *Maturitas* 2010;67:275–89.
22. Groff AA, Covington SN, Halverson LR, et al. Assessing the emotional needs of women with spontaneous premature ovarian failure. *Fertil Steril* 2005;83:1734–41.

12 Polycystic ovary syndrome

Polycystic ovary syndrome (PCOS) is a heterogeneous disorder that affects between 6 and 10% of women of reproductive age. The Rotterdam consensus on diagnostic criteria for PCOS was revised in 2003 to recognize the spectrum of clinical presentations with which this syndrome of ovarian dysfunction may present. PCOS remains a syndrome, and as such, no single diagnostic criterion is sufficient for a clinical diagnosis. It is therefore generally accepted that a patient should exhibit two out of three of the following findings *with the exclusion of other aetiologies*, such as congenital adrenal hyperplasia, androgen-secreting tumours, Cushing's syndrome, thyroid disease and hyperprolactinaemia:

- oligo- and/or anovulation
- clinical and/or biochemical signs of hyperandrogenism
- polycystic ovaries (12 or more cysts, 2–9 mm in diameter and/or increased ovarian volume of over 10 ml; see Figure 12.1).

The prevalence of PCOS will differ according to ethnic background. For example, women of South Asian origin may present at a younger age with more severe symptoms associated with PCOS.

Features of PCOS

The features of PCOS can be divided into clinical, metabolic and endocrine findings.

CLINICAL FEATURES

Menstrual abnormalities

Clinically, menstrual abnormalities are the cornerstone of the syndrome and menses are often infrequent representing an underlying problem of chronic anovulation. A direct complaint of infrequent periods is not usual and the patient is more likely to present indirectly in the infertility setting with sub-fertility secondary to anovulation. Menstrual cyclicity and flow tend to be very variable.

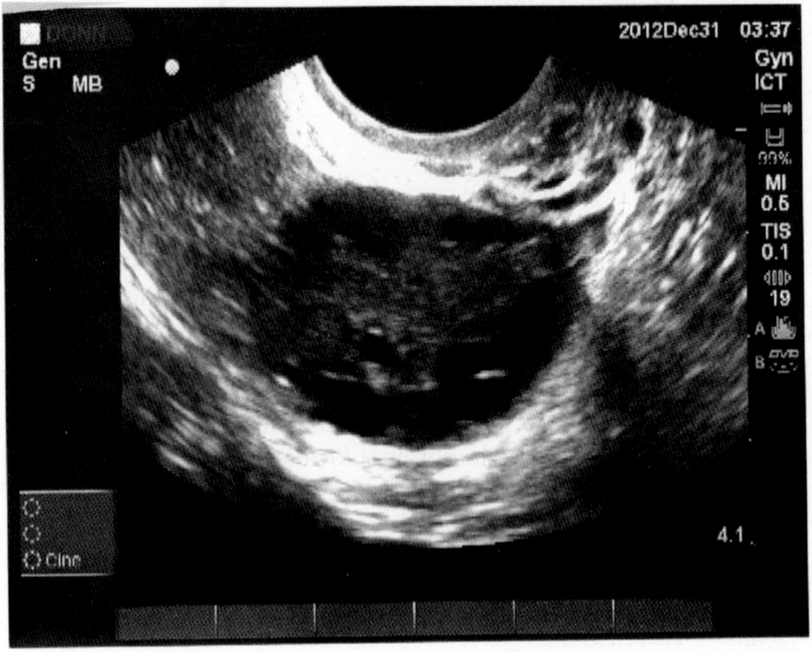

Figure 12.1 Ultrasound image of a polycystic ovary

Hyperandrogenism

It is thought that the primary clinical indicator of androgen excess is the presence of hirsutism. However, normative data for large populations are lacking and patients may have treated their hair growth prior to consultation. Additionally, assessment of hair distribution is often subjective and few physicians will use a standardized scoring method such as the Ferriman–Gallwey score. Other clinical indicators such as acne or alopecia may also represent an excessive androgenic state.

Biochemical hyperandrogenism is often evident and is discussed below in the section on investigations. However, a proportion of patients may not display any biochemical androgen abnormality.

Ultrasound polycystic ovaries

It is not unusual for an ultrasound report to comment on the appearance of an ovary being consistent with polycystic ovaries. A woman having polycystic ovaries in the absence of an ovulatory disorder or hyperandrogenism should not be considered as having PCOS. However, ultrasound findings are now considered as one of the criteria for diagnosing PCOS. The following situations should be considered when interpreting an ultrasound scan investigation of PCOS. If the woman is on the oral contraceptive pill, ultrasound features of ovarian morphology may be altered and therefore findings are of less value. If there is evidence of a dominant follicle, the scan should be repeated at a later date. If another ovarian pathology is found, then further investigations and referral should be arranged as appropriate.

ENDOCRINE AND METABOLIC FEATURES

Insulin resistance is a physiological condition where the natural hormone, insulin, becomes less effective at lowering blood sugars. Increased insulin resistance, defined as reduced glucose response to a given amount of insulin, is found in up to 50% of women with PCOS compared with 10 to 25% of the general population.[1] Obesity would appear to be an additive factor as obese PCOS women have been shown to have a decreased insulin sensitivity compared with non-obese women with PCOS.[2]

There is currently no readily available valid test for testing insulin resistance in clinical practice. A focus on the metabolic manifestations associated with increased insulin resistance is therefore used instead. Metabolic components often found in patients with PCOS include: centripetal obesity, hypertension, fasting hyperglycaemia and dyslipidaemia.

Impaired glucose tolerance may also be present and can be looked for using an oral glucose tolerance test. Impaired glucose tolerance is a major risk factor for developing diabetes and both conditions are associated with increased morbidity and mortality.

LH levels and its ratio to follicle-stimulating hormone (LH:FSH ratio) are both increased in PCOS as compared with controls. However, LH levels can be influenced by transient ovulation (normalizing levels), BMI and assay systems used. There are controversial suggestions that elevated LH levels have an independent detrimental effect on reproductive measures such as oocyte maturity, fertilization and increased miscarriage rates.[3] These suggestions have yet to be proved and, based on the lack of firm evidence regarding clinical effects of LH levels, LH levels may not be considered necessary for the clinical diagnosis of PCOS.

The majority of testosterone in the blood is tightly bound to sex hormone-binding globulin (SHBG) or to albumin. Only a small percentage is unbound and 'free' to bind tissue receptors to exert its effects.

Free testosterone would be a good marker of a person's androgen status; however, free testosterone is difficult to measure. The free androgen index (FAI) is the ratio used to determine abnormal androgen status. The ratio is the total testosterone level (bound and unbound) divided by the SHBG level, and then multiplying by a constant (usually 100).

Pathophysiology

The exact cause of PCOS is still not fully understood. It may be of use to consider a metabolic-ovarian-pituitary circuitry, which can be upset at many points. Disruption to this circuitry leads to the same functional endpoint of ovarian androgen excess and anovulation.

Weight loss has been shown to greatly improve insulin sensitivity.[4] Altered insulin receptor phosphorylation and hence impaired receptor activation has also been demonstrated in PCOS. Several studies have shown a positive correlation between fasting insulin levels and androgen levels. Whether hyperandrogenism results from hyperinsulinaemia or vice versa remains an ongoing debate and more research is required to answer this question. It has been shown that removal of ovarian androgen production, either surgically or by administration of a GnRH analogue, does not cause any change in hyperinsulinaemic state in PCOS.[5] However, some evidence has demonstrated a reduction of insulin resistance in response to anti-androgen therapy. It is generally accepted that the action of insulin augments ovarian androgen production by both a direct action upon ovarian insulin and insulin-like growth factor receptors and an indirect action, enhancing LH pulse amplitude.

Insulin will also inhibit hepatic synthesis of serum sex hormone-binding globulin (SHBG), which allows a greater amount of free androgen and oestrogen to be available.

The implication of insulin resistance leading to high androgen levels is that any intervention which can improve insulin sensitivity and reduce circulating insulin levels may relieve the hyperandrogenism.[6]

ANTI-MÜLLERIAN HORMONE (AMH)

AMH is produced in the granulosa cells of the ovaries, from 36 weeks of gestation until menopause, with the highest expression being in small antral follicles. AMH production gradually declines as follicles grow; once follicles reach a size at which they are dominant, AMH has largely disappeared. The removal of AMH from these larger follicles appears to be an important requirement for dominant follicle selection and progression to ovulation as AMH has an inhibitory role in the ovary, reducing both primordial follicle initiation and follicle sensitivity to FSH by inhibition of aromatase. In women with PCOS, serum levels of AMH are doubled and granulosa cell production is greatly increased. There appear to be two groups of women with PCOS, who can be distinguished by their AMH level. One group consists of those where the level is less elevated and reduces on ovulation induction, leading to a better response. The second group has high levels, which do not reduce with treatment and these women respond less well to induction of ovulation. Understanding the reason for the raised AMH in PCOS may give clues as to the mechanism of anovulation. To conclude, AMH appears to have a major inhibitory role during folliculogenesis, which may contribute to anovulation in PCOS.

Long-term health risks

Women with PCOS are at a three- to seven-fold elevated risk of developing type 2 diabetes and the health complications associated with this disease. Lifestyle influences and pharmacological intervention can influence this progression and screening for diabetes would therefore seem justified.

There is evidence demonstrating that PCOS is an independent risk factor for cardiovascular disease and, in particular, increased insulin resistance states have been linked to coronary heart disease. However, the relationship of PCOS with the incidence of coronary heart disease in later life is under, and clinicians should be aware that conventional cardiovascular risk calculators have not been devised for PCOS. Sleep apnoea is an independent cardiovascular risk and has been found to be more common in PCOS when compared with controls even when corrected for BMI.

The risk of endometrial cancer in women with PCOS is also thought to be elevated and chronic exposure to unopposed oestrogen through anovulation would provide a sound reasoning to explain this increased risk. However, epidemiological evidence to support this perceived link is so far limited.

Investigations

Pelvic ultrasound should be arranged to assess ovarian morphology and endometrial thickness. Transvaginal scans will provide a better assessment than transabdominal scans. It must be remembered that the finding of polycystic ovaries on an ultrasound scan is not, on its own, evidence of PCOS.

Biochemical evidence of a hyperandrogen state is best checked for via measurement of total testosterone and SHBG. If total testosterone levels exceed 5 nmol/l, referral for further investigations is warranted to exclude rare causes such as androgen-secreting tumours. Measurement of FAI is useful, as a raised level in the presence of a normal total testosterone is a common finding in PCOS.

Prolactin levels should be measured in oligo-/amenorrhoeic women to exclude a prolactinoma; however, levels of prolactin are often in the upper range of normality or slightly elevated in women with PCOS. A fasting glucose should be organised to exclude impaired glucose tolerance and/or diabetes. Because insulin resistance is greater in the obese population, a glucose tolerance test should be arranged if the BMI is over 30kg/m^2, but this threshold may be lowered if additional risk factors such as ethnicity or family history are present.

LH and FSH are not very useful in the diagnosis of PCOS. If they are to be measured, blood should be taken, if possible, during days 1–3 of the menstrual cycle. Oestradiol levels are unhelpful in making a diagnosis.

Treatment

Women diagnosed with PCOS should be informed of the possible long-term risks to health that are associated with their condition. They should be advised regarding weight control and exercise as this forms the cornerstone of treatment. Significant weight loss has been shown to result in spontaneous resumption of ovulation and improvement in infertility,[7] increased SHBG and reduced basal levels of insulin.[4] Achieving weight loss is very hard for these patients and many women may experience frustration in their attempts to lose weight, leading to problems of low mood and/or low self-esteem.

Dietary advice about healthy eating would usually include reducing fat and sugar intake while increasing consumption of fruit, vegetables and complex carbohydrates. Referral to a dietitian can be helpful to obtain individually tailored dietary advice. Diet is important but an increase in physical activity is essential. A target of 30 minutes of brisk exercise a day is required to maintain health but, in order to lose weight, the patient may well have to target a regime of more than 1 hour of exercise each day.

Anti-obesity drugs may help with weight loss. Both orlistat and sibutramine have been shown to be effective in PCOS, but monitoring of efficacy is important. Only orlistat is available in the UK. Both agents have been shown to improve insulin resistance, lipid profile and glycaemic control. Orlistat has additionally been shown to reduce blood pressure and testosterone. Metformin has been shown to aid with modest weight loss, although, importantly, this has not been confirmed in randomised controlled trials. Metformin's possible health benefits are in improving insulin resistance and hyperandrogenism, restoring menstrual cycle and possibly fertility. Gastrointestinal adverse effects often reduce patient compliance; taking tablets with food and starting with a low dose and gradually building up over 2–3 weeks can reduce these. Metformin is not licensed for treatment of PCOS but, when used, the target dose is around 500 mg three times a day or 850 mg twice daily.

After advice and help about weight loss, the management of a woman with PCOS should be targeted towards her individual problems.

MENSTRUAL IRREGULARITY

If contraception is required, the easiest method of controlling a menstrual cycle is with the use of a low-dose oral contraceptive pill. Alternatively, a progestogen may be used to induce a withdrawal bleed every 1–3 months to prevent unopposed oestrogen, which is prevalent in PCOS, leading to endometrial hyperplasia. The Mirena intrauterine system may also be of benefit in this role. If amenorrhoea is persistent and endometrial thickening is evident on ultrasound scan, an endometrial biopsy should be taken.

INFERTILITY

Ovulation induction can be achieved with clomiphene citrate (50–100 mg) from days 2 to 6 of a natural or induced menses. Ovulation can be achieved in up to 80% of women; however, pregnancy will occur only in about 40%. Ultrasound monitoring is advisable to try and reduce the 10% risk of multiple pregnancy. Once an ovulation dose has been achieved, the cumulative pregnancy rates will increase for up to 10–12 cycles.[8] However, clomiphene is licensed only for use for up to 6 months in the UK and an extension of this period should involve careful counselling about the possible increase in ovarian cancer rates. Metformin has an accumulating body of evidence demonstrating its safety in use for PCOS and also in pregnancy. However, it is not licensed in the UK for use in women who are not diabetic. There is a small amount of evidence suggesting that metformin may reduce miscarriage rates and the development of gestational diabetes in women with PCOS, but the evidence is not strong. Despite the common use of insulin-sensitizing agents, the RCOG does not currently recommend the use of metformin in pregnancy.

Women who are resistant to anti-estrogens may benefit from either parenteral gonadotrophins or laparoscopic ovarian diathermy. Cumulative conception and live birth rates after 6 months for gonadotrophin therapies are 62% and 54%, respectively. Women with PCOS are very sensitive to exogenous hormones and regimes will start with a low dose. Women with PCOS are also at risk of developing ovarian hyperstimulation syndrome and treatment should be suspended if three or more mature follicles develop. Ovarian drilling is not associated with multiple pregnancies or ovarian hyperstimulation syndrome and live birth rates are similar to those achieved with gonadotrophin therapy, particularly in slim women.

HYPERANDROGENISM

Hirsutism is a very distressing symptom for a woman with PCOS but unfortunately it is difficult to treat. Drug therapies may take 6–9 months to provide any benefit for hirsutism and use of cosmetic techniques is pragmatic and effective. Physical treatments include electrolysis, laser therapy, waxing and bleaching or eflornithine cream. Electrolysis is a long-lasting treatment but is time consuming, painful and expensive and regrowth is not uncommon. More recently, the use of different types of laser techniques has showed promise in many patients if appropriately selected (dark hair on fair skin is best).

Eflornithine is a topical treatment for facial hirsutism and may be used in conjunction with hormonal treatments while waiting for them to work. Eflornithine works by inhibiting the ornithine decarboxylase enzyme in hair follicles and improvement should be evident within 8 weeks.

Medical anti-androgen therapies include the use of cyproterone acetate, spironolactone, finastride and flutamide. Transplacental passage of anti-androgens may disturb development of the male fetus and adequate contraception is therefore essential. Finastride and flutamide are rarely used in the UK and are no more effective than cyproterone acetate. Cyproterone acetate is commonly used in combination with ethinyl estradiol, often in the form of Dianette, an oral contraceptive pill. Improvement in acne with Dianette will take 4–6 months and improvement in hirsutism will take longer. Cyproterone acetate can rarely cause liver damage and liver function tests should be checked after 6 months and then annually.

References

1. The Rotterdam ESHRE/ARSM-Sponsored PCOS consensus workshop group. Revised 2003 consensus on diagnostic criteria and long-term health risks related to polycystic ovary syndrome (PCOS). *Hum Reprod* 2004;19:41–7.
2. Morales AJ, Laughlin GA, Bützow T, Maheshwari H, Baumann G, Yen SS. Insulin, somatotropic, and luteinizing hormone axes in lean and obese women with polycystic ovary syndrome: common and distinct features. *J Clin Endocrinol Metab* 1996;81:2854–64.
3. Tarlatzis BC, Grimbizis G, Pournaropoulos F, et al. The prognostic value of basal luteinizing hormone:follicle-stimulating hormone ratio in the treatment of patients with PCOS by assisted reproduction techniques. *Hum Reprod* 1995;10:2545–9.
4. Huber-Buchholz MM, Carey DG, Norman RJ. Restoration of reproductive potential by lifestyle modification in obese polycystic ovary syndrome: role of insulin sensitivity and luteinizing hormone. *J Clin Endocrinol Metab* 1999;84:1470–4.
5. Tsilchorozidou T, Overton C, Conway G. The pathophysiology of polycystic ovary syndrome. *Clin Endocrinol (Oxf)* 2004;60:1–17.
6. Velazquez EM, Mendoza SG, Wang P, Glueck CJ. Metformin therapy is associated with a decrease in plasma plasminogen activator inhibitor-1, lipoprotein(a), and immunoreactive insulin levels in patients with the polycystic ovary syndrome. *Metabolism* 1997;46:454–7.
7. Crosignani PG, Colombo M, Vegetti W, Somigliana E, Gessati A, Ragni G. Overweight and obese anovulatory patients with polycystic ovaries: parallel improvements in anthropometric indices, ovarian physiology and fertility rate induced by diet. *Hum Reprod* 2003;18:1928–32.
8. Kousta E, White DM, Franks S. Modern use of clomiphene citrate in induction of ovulation. *Hum Reprod Update* 1997;3:359–65.

Further reading

Royal College of Obstetricians and Gynaecologists. *Long-term Consequences of Polycystic Ovary Syndrome*. Green-top Guideline no. 33. London: RCOG; 2007 [http://www.rcog.org.uk/womens-health/clinical-guidance/long-term-consequences-polycystic-ovary-syndrome-green-top-33].

13 Premenstrual syndrome

Premenstrual syndrome (PMS) or PMT is a common problem which can markedly interfere with normal life.[1–4] It is frustrating for both patients and doctors as there is no biological marker and severity can fluctuate from cycle to cycle.[5] Most women have one or more emotional or physical symptoms in the premenstrual phase of the menstrual cycle. Although these symptoms are usually mild, 5%–8% of women have moderate or severe symptoms. Premenstrual dysphoric disorder (PMDD) is a more severe variant that includes at least one affective symptom. DSM-IV criteria require five or more physical and behavioural symptoms from a pre-specified list to be recorded using a diary.[6] The diagnosis of PMDD stipulates:

- the presence of at least five luteal-phase symptoms (Box 13.1), at least one of which must be a mood symptom such as anxiety or tension, depressed mood, affect lability, or persistent anger and irritability;
- two cycles of daily charting to confirm the timing of symptoms; and
- evidence of functional impairment.

Symptoms must not be the exacerbation of another psychiatric condition. The International Society for Premenstrual Disorders (ISPMD) has made recommendations for a new classification with core (the typical, pure or reference disorders associated with spontaneous ovulatory menstrual cycles) and variant premenstrual disorders (such as symptoms of an underlying psychological or somatic disorder significantly worsening premenstrually).[7]

Aetiology

PMS is related to cyclical ovarian function as it is absent before the menarche and is cured by the menopause. However, the way in which ovarian steroids provoke luteal symptoms which may start at different times (just after ovulation, or just before menstruation) are unclear. The importance of progesterone compared with oestrogen in triggering

BOX 13.1 CLINICAL CRITERIA FOR PMDD

DSM-IV criteria for PMDD[6] require at least five of 11 symptoms during the luteal phase. Symptoms must resolve soon after menses start and be absent after menses. At least one symptom must be among the first four listed:

- Depressed mood
- Significant anxiety
- Affective lability
- Persistent anger or irritability
- Decreased interest in usual activities
- Concentration difficulty
- Lethargy
- Change in eating habits
- Insomnia or hypersomnia
- Sense of being overwhelmed
- Physical symptoms (breast tenderness, headaches, bloating, weight gain).

The symptoms severely interfere with usual activities and relationships. Symptoms should not be associated with another psychiatric disorder.

Evidence must be recorded in a diary for at least two symptomatic menstrual cycles.

symptoms is also uncertain. Mood change reported by postmenopausal women taking sequential hormone replacement therapy suggests that progesterone, rather than oestrogen, is responsible for inducing dysphoria. Furthermore, oestrogen exerts an antidepressant effect in women with perimenopausal depression. On the other hand, oestradiol can provoke PMS-like complaints and luteal administration of an oestrogen antagonist reduces premenstrual mastalgia.

Evidence suggests that women with and without PMS do not differ with respect to the production of gonadal steroids, indicating that PMS might instead be associated with enhanced responsiveness to normal, fluctuating concentrations of these hormones.

The results of twin and family studies suggest that PMS is a heritable disorder. Genotypic differences are likely to mediate a differential behavioural response to gonadal steroids. An association has been found between allelic variants in the oestrogen receptor alpha gene and PMS. Other possible risk factors for PMS are high BMI, stress and traumatic events.

Neurotransmitters must be involved in PMS as mood changes are important symptoms. The most important candidate is serotonin and indeed selective serotonin reuptake inhibitors (SSRIs) are effective treatments (see below). In addition, oestrogen has antidopaminergic properties and progesterone modulates gamma aminobutyric acid, the neurotransmitter involved in emotional control.

Assessment

It is essential to listen to the woman and take her complaint seriously. She may have asked other doctors for help in the past without success and may be aggrieved that she has been dismissed. Essential questions to ask are:

- What are the symptoms?
- How long has this been a problem?
- What is your menstrual history?
- What contraception is being used?
- Is there a past history of psychiatric problems or traumatic events?

The diagnosis of PMS and PMDD requires daily charting of symptoms over two or three menstrual cycles because of the variability of symptoms. Various scoring systems and diaries have been developed for this purpose, such as the Daily Record of Severity of Problems and the Moos Menstrual Distress Questionnaire.[8,9] While women may be reluctant to participate in such an exercise, perceiving it as a way of delaying treatment, it is essential to distinguish between:

- true PMS/PMDD
- premenstrual exacerbation of an underlying psychiatric disorder
- a condition with no relation to the menstrual cycle.

Treatment

Understanding the woman's problems is essential and indeed may be the most therapeutic option. The one consistent factor in randomized controlled trials on any of the PMS treatments is the very high placebo response – about 60% improvement. Despite lack of specific evidence, lifestyle modifications and exercise are first-line recommendations for all women with PMS/PMDD and may be all that is needed to treat mild to moderate symptoms.

SSRIs

SSRIs have been proven safe and effective for the treatment of PMDD.[10,11,12] The response rate is usually 60%–90% for active treatment versus 30%–40% for placebo. They can be recommended as first-line agents when pharmacotherapy is warranted in women with severe mood symptoms. SSRIs are approved for PMDD in the USA, Canada and Australia, but not in Europe. The European Agency for the Evaluation of Medicinal Products withdrew the existing licence for fluoxetine in four European countries including the UK. Currently fluoxetine, controlled-release paroxetine and sertraline are the only Food and Drug Administration-approved agents for this indication. The beneficial effect of SSRIs for PMS begins rapidly, rendering intermittent luteal treatment a feasible alternative to continuous therapy. Some women find it more acceptable to take antidepressants intermittently, rather than feeling 'addicted' to them. However intermittent use is less effective than continuous dosing.

Health professionals must be prepared to encounter patients with PMS who are considering pregnancy. SSRIs have been associated with significant risks of major malformation, particularly cardiac defects, and behaviour syndromes when used during pregnancy.[13,14] Therefore, patients should be advised of the reproductive safety of these medications and the importance of balancing the risk versus the benefits on an individual basis.

HORMONAL INTERVENTIONS

Suppression of ovulation using hormonal therapies is an alternative approach to treating PMDD when SSRIs or second-line psychotropic agents are ineffective.[1,2,3,15] However, adverse effects for the majority of strategies limit their use. Since PMS is caused by cyclical ovarian function, ablating the cycle by various means may be effective. If this is not effective, the woman does not have PMS. While GnRH agonists are effective there are concerns about the safety of long-term use as they induce a medical menopause with symptoms such as bone loss, although this is significantly reduced by co-administration of HRT. Surgical bilateral oophorectomy is also effective, but is irreversible and should be considered only as the solution to a desperate situation.[3] Although no research evidence is available to support this, administration of a GnRH agonist for 2 to 3 months before surgery will show the patient the probable effect of removing the ovaries and could inform her decision.

The synthetic androgen and gonadotropin inhibitor danazol, when administered at doses that block ovulation, is effective for PMS.

However, hirsutism and other androgenic side effects and risk of teratogenicity preclude its long-term use.[1,2]

To suppress ovulation, 100 microgram oestrogen patches are effective, but the number of studies is limited.[3] Doses are usually higher than are those required for HRT. Unless the patient has had a hysterectomy, she will need to be given progestogen to prevent endometrial hyperplasia. This could result in re-stimulation of PMS in some patients, unless it is administered with a levonorgestrel intrauterine device.

If the woman needs contraception, continuous combined oral contraception should help, as does [in some cases] the levonorgestrel intrauterine device, but there are few placebo-controlled studies. One oral contraceptive containing drospirenone as the progestogen which exerts anti-aldosterone and anti-androgen effects appears promising but more data are awaited.

The role of progesterone is uncertain and a systematic review, which found only two trials suitable for inclusion, concluded: 'We could not say that progesterone helped women with PMS, nor that it was ineffective'.[16] There is no good evidence about the role of depot progestogens.

OTHER PHARMACOTHERAPY

Anxiolytics, spironolactone and non-steroidal anti-inflammatory drugs can be used as supportive care to relieve symptoms. Most studies assessing the therapeutic effect of vitamin B6 (pyridoxine) in PMS have several methodological limitations, including lack of prospective ratings. It can cause neuropathy in excessive doses.[1,2,3]

COGNITIVE BEHAVIOURAL THERAPY

The aim of cognitive behavioural therapy (CBT) is to improve coping strategies. A systematic review has concluded that 'Low quality evidence from randomized trials suggests that cognitive behavioural therapy may have important beneficial effects in managing symptoms associated with premenstrual syndrome.'[17]

ALTERNATIVE AND COMPLEMENTARY THERAPIES

Herbal and vitamin supplementation and complementary and alternative medicine have been evaluated for use in PMS/PMDD, producing unclear or conflicting results.[18,19,20] A wide variety of products are used: oil of evening primrose, St John's Wort, chasteberry, pollen, saffron and Chinese herbal medicines. More controlled clinical trials are needed to determine their safety and efficacy and potential for drug interactions. Oil of evening primrose oil may help breast tenderness. St John's Wort is really a SSRI.

Conclusion

Dealing with premenstrual syndrome is a clinical challenge as it is a socially acceptable diagnosis which may used as a calling card for psychological or psychiatric disorders. It is important to assess carefully over several cycles and explain there is no diagnostic blood test. Treatment is symptom based and will have to be used for many years until the menopause and will have to take into account the woman's reproductive goals.

References

1. Map of Medicine Premenstrual syndrome [http://healthguides.mapofmedicine.com/choices/map/menstrual_cycle_irregularities_and_post_menopausal_bleeding_pmb_7.html].
2. O'Brien S, Rapkin A, Dennerstein L et al. Diagnosis and management of premenstrual disorders. *BMJ* 2011;342;1297–303.
3. BMJ Point of Care/Best Practice: Premenstrual syndrome and dysphoric disorder [http://bestpractice.bmj.com/best-practice/welcome.html].
4. Royal College of Obstetricians and Gynaecologists. *Management of Premenstrual Syndrome*. Green-top Guideline No. 48. London: RCOG; 2007.
5. Potter J, Bouyer J, Trussell J, Moreau C. Premenstrual syndrome prevalence and fluctuation over time: results from a French population-based survey. *J Womens Health (Larchmt)* 2009;18:31–9.
6. American Psychiatric Association. *Diagnostic and Statistical Manual of Mental Disorders – DSM-IV*. 4th ed. Washington DC: American Psychiatric Association; 1994.
7. O'Brien PM, Bäckström T, Brown C, et al. Towards a consensus on diagnostic criteria, measurement and trial design of the premenstrual disorders: the ISPMD Montreal consensus. *Arch Womens Ment Health* 2011;14:13–21.
8. Borenstein JE, Dean BB, Yonkers KA, Endicott J. Using the daily record of severity of problems as a screening instrument for premenstrual syndrome. *Obstet Gynecol* 2007;109:1068–75.
9. Ross C, Coleman G, Stojanovska C. Factor structure of the modified Moos Menstrual Distress Questionnaire: assessment of prospectively reported follicular, menstrual and premenstrual symptomatology. *J Psychosom Obstet Gynaecol* 2003;24:163–74.
10. Landén M, Nissbrandt H, Allgulander C, Sörvik K, Ysander C, Eriksson E. Placebo-controlled trial comparing intermittent and continuous

paroxetine in premenstrual dysphoric disorder. *Neuropsychopharmacology* 2007;32:153–61.
11. Shah NR, Jones JB, Aperi J, Shemtov R, Karne A, Borenstein J. Selective serotonin reuptake inhibitors for premenstrual syndrome and premenstrual dysphoric disorder: a meta-analysis. *Obstet Gynecol* 2008;111:1175–82.
12. Steiner M, Ravindran AV, LeMelledo JM, et al. Luteal phase administration of paroxetine for the treatment of premenstrual dysphoric disorder: a randomized, double-blind, placebo-controlled trial in Canadian women. *J Clin Psychiatry* 2008;69:991–8.
13. Tuccori M, Testi A, Antonioli L, et al. Safety concerns associated with the use of serotonin reuptake inhibitors and other serotonergic/noradrenergic antidepressants during pregnancy: a review. *Clin Ther* 2009;31:1426–53.
14. Kieler H, Artama M, Engeland A, et al. Selective serotonin reuptake inhibitors during pregnancy and risk of persistent pulmonary hypertension in the newborn: population based cohort study from the five Nordic countries. *BMJ* 2011;344:d8012.
15. Lopez LM, Kaptein A, Helmerhorst FM. Oral contraceptives containing drospirenone for premenstrual syndrome. *Cochrane Database Syst Rev* 2008;(1):CD006586.
16. Ford O, Lethaby A, Mol B, Roberts H. Progesterone for premenstrual syndrome. *Cochrane Database Syst Rev* 2006;(4):CD003415.
17. Busse JW, Montori VM, Krasnik C, Patelis-Siotis I, Guyatt GH. Psychological intervention for premenstrual syndrome: a meta-analysis of randomized controlled trials. *Psychother Psychosom* 2009;78:6–15.
18. Agha-Hosseini M, Kashani L, Aleyaseen A, et al. Crocus sativus L. (saffron) in the treatment of premenstrual syndrome: a double-blind, randomised and placebo-controlled trial. *BJOG* 2008;115:515–19.
19. Gerhardsen G, Hansen AV, Killi M, Fornitz GG, Pedersen F, Roos SB. The efficacy of Femal in women with premenstrual syndrome: a randomised, double-blind, parallel-group, placebo-controlled, multicentre study. *Adv Ther* 2008;25:595–607.
20. Jing Z, Yang X, Ismail KM, Chen X, Wu T. Chinese herbal medicine for premenstrual syndrome. *Cochrane Database Syst Rev* 2009;(1):CD006414.

Index